Melissa Rañoa '02

Melissa Rañoa '02

LatinaBeauty

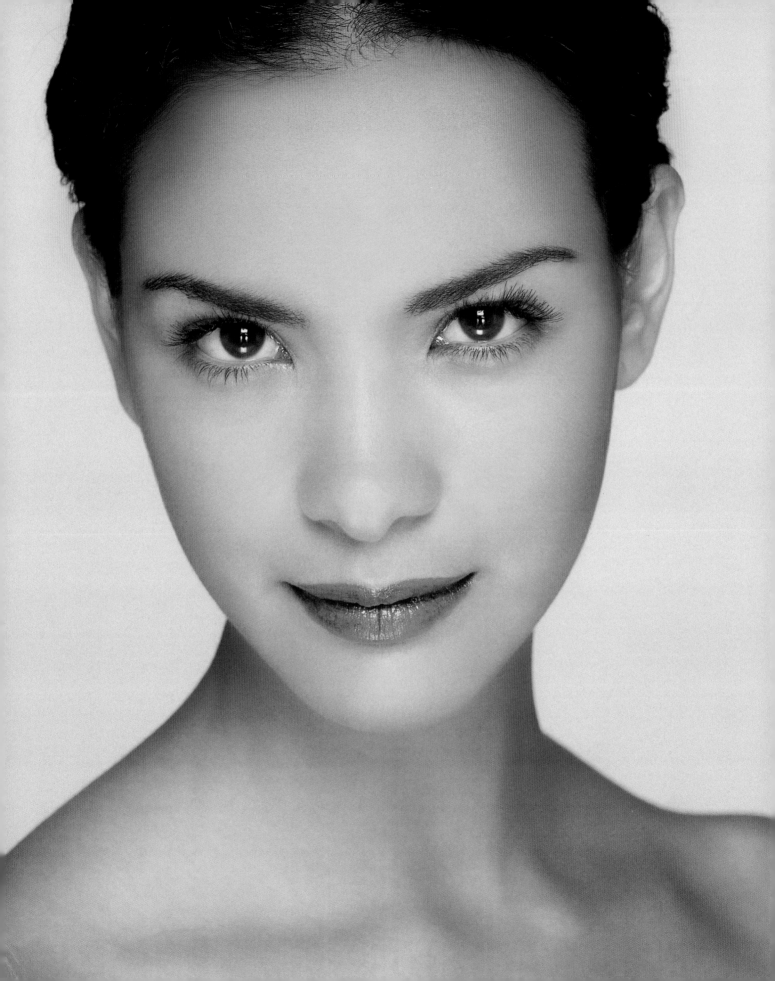

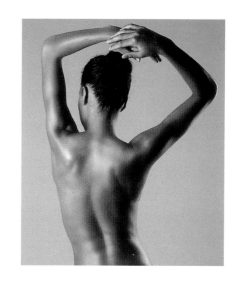

A Get-Gorgeous Guide
for Every *Mujer*

Latina Beauty

The Editors of *Latina* Magazine and Belén Aranda-Alvarado

with a Foreword by Daisy Fuentes

A Welcome Book

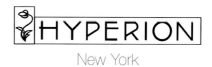
HYPERION
New York

Contents

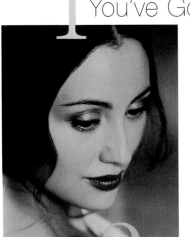

1 You've Got *Ese Algo*...........p.9

Redefine what it means to be beautiful by starting from within.
Give yourself permission to express your true *belleza*.

2 About Base...........p.23
Base, Powder, and Concealer

Get the shade that enhances—not masks—your beautiful skin.
Selecting, applying, and maximizing your color choices.

3 Blush & Pout...........p.39

Your lips speak volumes, so match the look to your mood. Find
the always-right color for your cheeks and master bronzer basics.

4 Luminous *Ojos*...........p.55

Beautiful eyes in five minutes flat, make the many shades of
brown eyes even more alluring, and explore different looks.

5 Silky, Curly, Sexy, Straight...........p.77
Your Crowning Glory

Stick with what nature gave you or experiment with what some nurturing
can do. Tips for every hair texture, length, and color.

6 Get the Glow...........p.101
Sensual, Smooth Skin

Get sexy with these pointers for healthy, touchable *piel*.
Then get ready to bare it all.

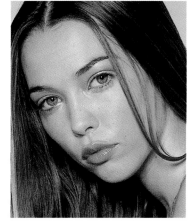

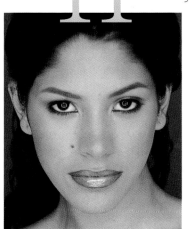

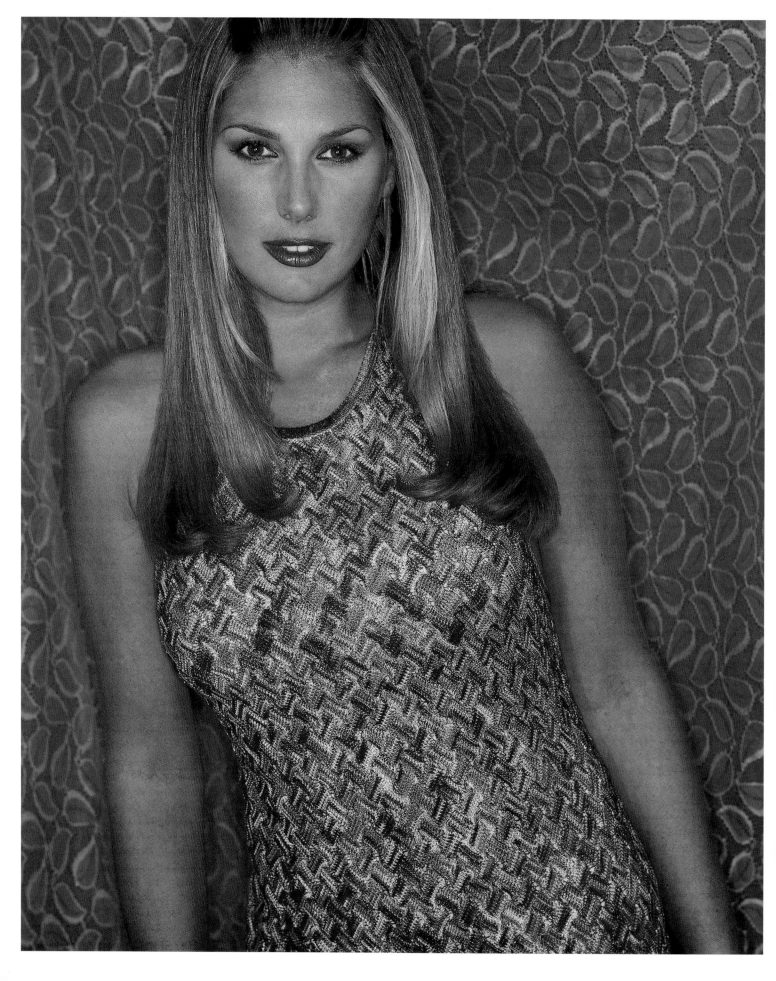

Foreword

THE THING I LIKE MOST ABOUT MYSELF IS MY BRAIN. MY BEST ASSETS ARE MY HEART AND my ability to listen and to love. My butt is cute, too. And for me, that is what beauty is all about—expressing that inner beauty, having a strong, clear mind, but also appreciating and having fun with your outer features.

My definition of what it means to be truly beautiful begins from within. About six years ago, I started to feel more confident about myself. I made a point of not allowing myself to be surrounded by jealousy, envy, or insecurity. Making that conscious choice allowed me to start enjoying the beauty that is all around us. I now make a point of filling myself with beautiful thoughts, of reading beautiful books, of being with people who have beautiful things to say. Beauty is an atmosphere you choose to live in.

From that point on, it became much easier to enjoy the accoutrements of outer beauty; it was that much more enjoyable to get my hair done, to have a manicure and pedicure, and to relish being sexy and glam. The makeup, the hair, the nails—these are things that make being a woman so much fun.

Of course, we have all had our beauty disasters, and I am no exception. The '80s—the entire decade—were my beauty nightmare. The huge hair, the tanning-booth skin—yeah, I did it all. At least I can say now that I was willing to experiment with a lot of different looks . . .

But through all the different hair styles and new makeup trends, I still know what I like best about me and where I find my true beauty. I may be the only *cubana* who didn't use Mirta de Perales hair products growing up, but I know what makes Latinas so beautiful. With our myriad of hair textures, our skin that ranges from alabaster to deep chocolate to sexy, smooth honey, what makes us beautiful is an inner spirit, and we all have part of it. I call it the salsa gene. Expressing our salsa gene is the best thing we can do for ourselves. It gives us permission to be as beautiful as we can be. It also defines what Latina beauty is: not a look, but an attitude.

—DAISY FUENTES

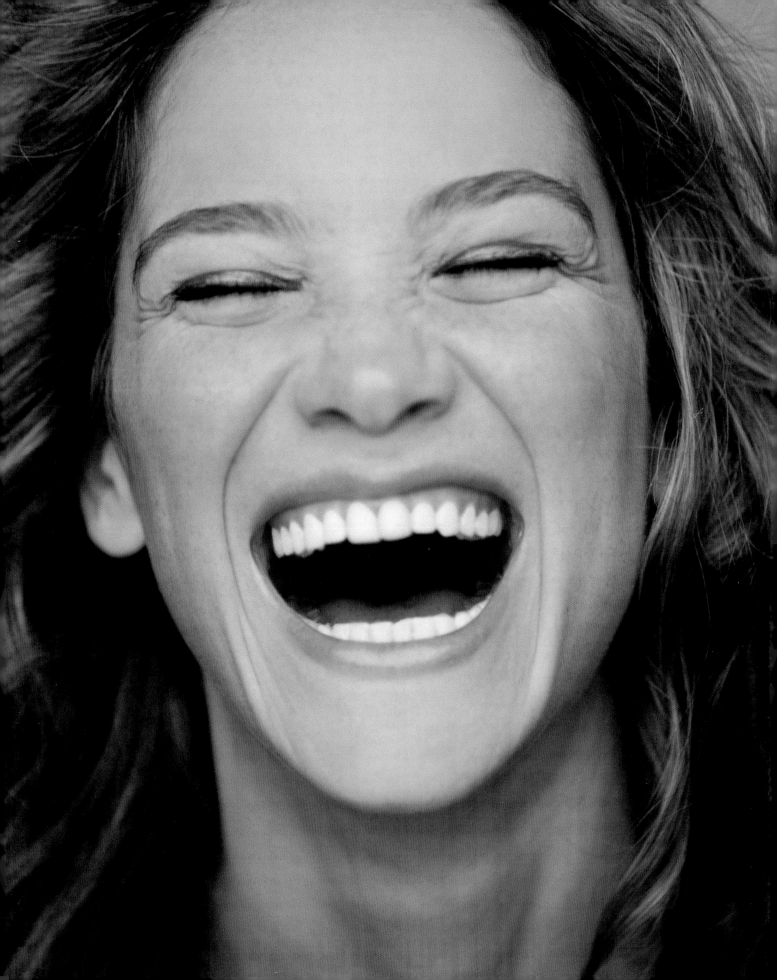

You've Got *Ese Algo*

TRUE BEAUTY COMES FROM WITHIN. IT'S NOT ABOUT THE MAKEUP YOU APPLY OR THE WAY you style your hair. Instead, beauty is energy, an attitude that is exciting, dynamic, and attractive. We know this is true because we see it every day; in our families, in our communities, and among our *comadres*, we spot these women. They may not have the blond hair and blue eyes of most super-models—much less the six-foot height or 36-25-36 measurements popular culture idolizes—and they can be any age, often far older than the typical 20-year-old beauty queen. Yet they still radiate *ese algo*. They look fabulous and love the life they are living. Beyond typical physical beauty, *tienen algo* that reveals they know what they are about and what they hope to accomplish in their lives. Even if they don't have all of life's questions completely figured out, these women are excited at the prospect of finding the answers eventually.

Ese algo comes in so many different forms, with so many different names. Some call it spirituality; some call it self-confidence; some people just call it a glow. But the bottom line is that this inner beauty is something we all have. It's our birthright as Latina women. Our mothers and their mothers before them worked hard and made tremendous sacrifices to bring us where we are today. We have pride, a beautiful culture, and a rich history we can access and express. In every way, we have *ese algo*. We are amazing women, *hermanas*.

But it's hard to emanate *ese algo* when, say, the baby has colic, you need sleep, and you have a big presentation at the office the next day. Yet whatever difficulties we experience in our daily lives, we owe it to ourselves to harness this energy, to articulate it, and to make it what it is meant to be: a fountain of empowerment fueled by the intuition that leads us to assert our best selves. The steps we take and principles we live by allow us to do this to our fullest.

*"One thing that makes a woman beautiful is the certainty
that she is beautiful. Like a woman who uses her confidence to
express herself—if you think that you're beautiful, then you are."*
—ISABEL ALLENDE

1. Give Yourself Permission
to **Love Your Life**

LOVING YOUR LIFE IS NOT ABOUT SETTLING FOR OR BEING SATISFIED with mediocrity. It means loving who you are, where you come from, and where you are going. If you love your life, you love the process and the journey life is—the lessons that become blessings, the small changes that become fundamental shifts, the uncertainties and chaos that you face, manage, and overcome every day. Ultimately, what loving your life gives you is a sense of inner peace. Inner peace is like knowledge and an education—something no one can take away. You can be stripped of money, title, possessions, even loved ones. But inner peace is a jewel that never dulls.

Ese algo also brings with it the recognition that we have a divine imperative to take care of ourselves from within and to express our inner and outer beauty. Most of us grew up with parents who made enormous sacrifices so we could have a better life. We honor their choices and their sacrifices when we take advantage of the opportunities that lie before us.

What *ese algo* shows us as well is that putting forth the time and effort to feel and look our best has a ripple effect: It makes us better mothers, wives, friends, and leaders. When we pause to regroup, refocus, and reenergize, we give a gift to ourselves, which makes us in turn more able to give to others. You owe this to yourself, and your *comunidad* needs it from you as well.

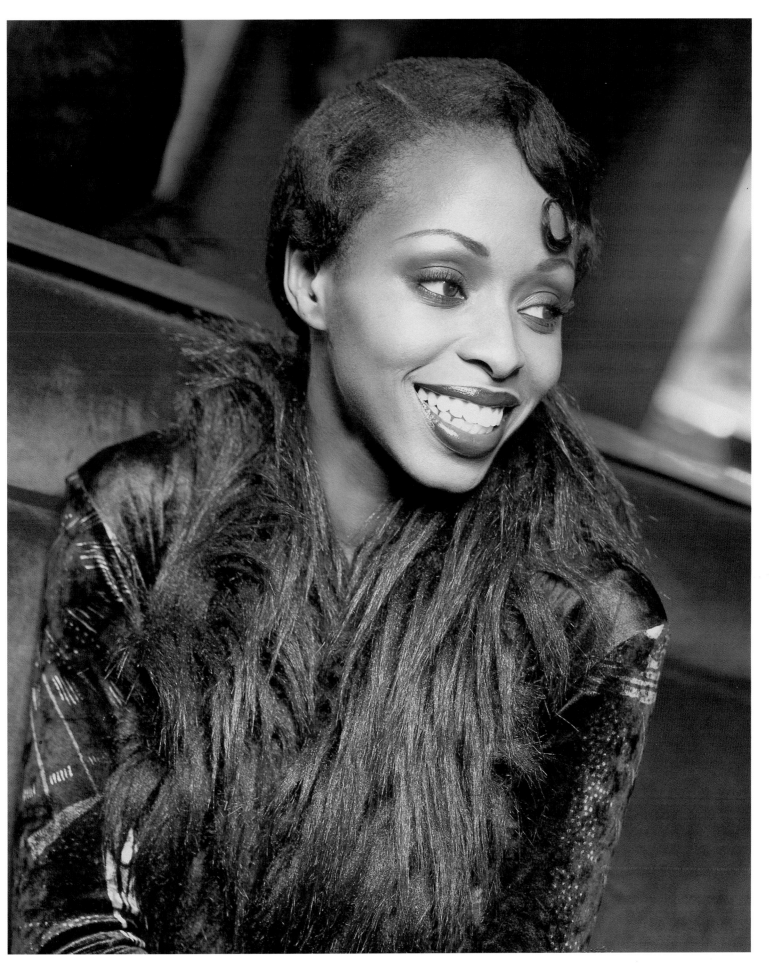

2. Surround Yourself with **Positive People** and **Positive Relationships**

AGUANTANDO, OR ENDURING—SOMETHING LATINAS KNOW A LOT about and do a little too much of—became, over time, a powerful stereotype of Hispanic women. But the quiet, passive, long-suffering Latina is a thing of the past. And for many of us, it's a stereotype that never even applied. Most of our mothers were *sin pelos en la lengua* and could keep us in line with just one look. *Aguantando* does have its positive side, however; it has enabled our women to survive—even thrive—amid difficult circumstances, while maintaining the tenacity to keep going forward and maintain faith, no matter what.

Even if your mother fits the *mujer que aguanta todo* stereotype, does this mean you should forget to give her credit for the amazing things she has done with her life? Giving birth to a fabulous, intelligent modern Latina like you is just one of her accomplishments. What about how she worked (in or outside the home), kept the family together, and passed on to you a sense of your *herencia* and *tradición*? Even women who appeared to fit the stereotype defied it in their own ways. Your mother wasn't a victim, and you certainly aren't going to be.

In any case, the second thing you need to do to recognize your inner beauty and to seize upon the exhilarating power of *ese algo* is to stop *aguantando*, and to do so immediately. What we usually end up *aguantando* is relationships or relationship patterns that have outgrown their usefulness in our lives.

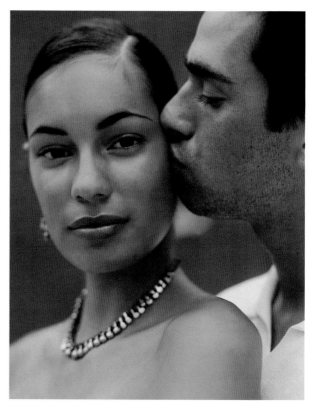

Surround yourself with people who are positive, not only about themselves and their lives but about you: people who see your potential and expect you to live up to it, people who are going places and doing things—people, ultimately, like yourself. Folks who whine about their lives or, worse, have *envidia* toward those who have what they want are like a weight that brings you down and holds you back. Wearing a charm to protect against *mal de ojo* won't do a thing if you insist on spending time with this brand of individual.

Certain relationships that outgrow their usefulness may be with people you can't simply discard from your life, like family members or coworkers. If this is the case, the thing to do is to alter the relationship pattern, because the chances of you actually being able to overhaul the relationship are slim. What you can change is how you react to their negativity. Minimize your interactions with these people, and do not allow anger, fear, or sadness to rule your behavior when you are with them. Eventually, you will come to realize that *aguantando* is a choice, and you are the one making it. (Of course, a little *mal de ojo* charm never hurt either.)

3. **Educate** Yourself

PERHAPS THE MOST EFFECTIVE WAY TO MAINtain *ese algo* is to get an education. Working at what you love and are passionate about is vital to facilitating *ese algo*, yet a college degree, while one of the best routes, is not the only ticket there. We all know college graduates who still don't know what they want from their lives, much less from themselves, and we all know incredible *mujeres* who have constructed remarkable lives without so much as a high school diploma. In all cases, what separates women with *ese algo* from women without it is intellectual curiosity.

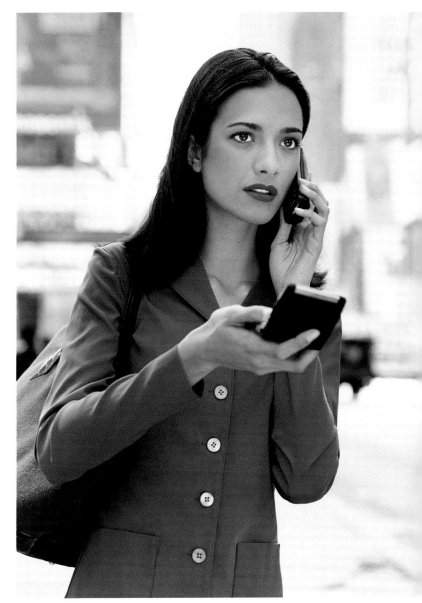

A college degree is the socially accepted pronouncement that you possess this important trait. But being a voracious reader, taking classes in subjects that interest you, having the ability to discuss any number of topics with any number of people, not being afraid to ask questions—these are all ways to have, cultivate, and express intellectual curiosity.

The *comadre* with no high school education who raises a healthy, happy family, starts a business, or becomes a community leader has at some point decided what she is passionate about. From that first decision, she went on to learn more about her interest and applied that knowledge to her goals on a daily basis. These were the ways in which she educated herself. Her education was a mix of experience, persistence, and trial and error

Make a commitment to learn more, read more, ask more. That is the best way to actually *do* more.

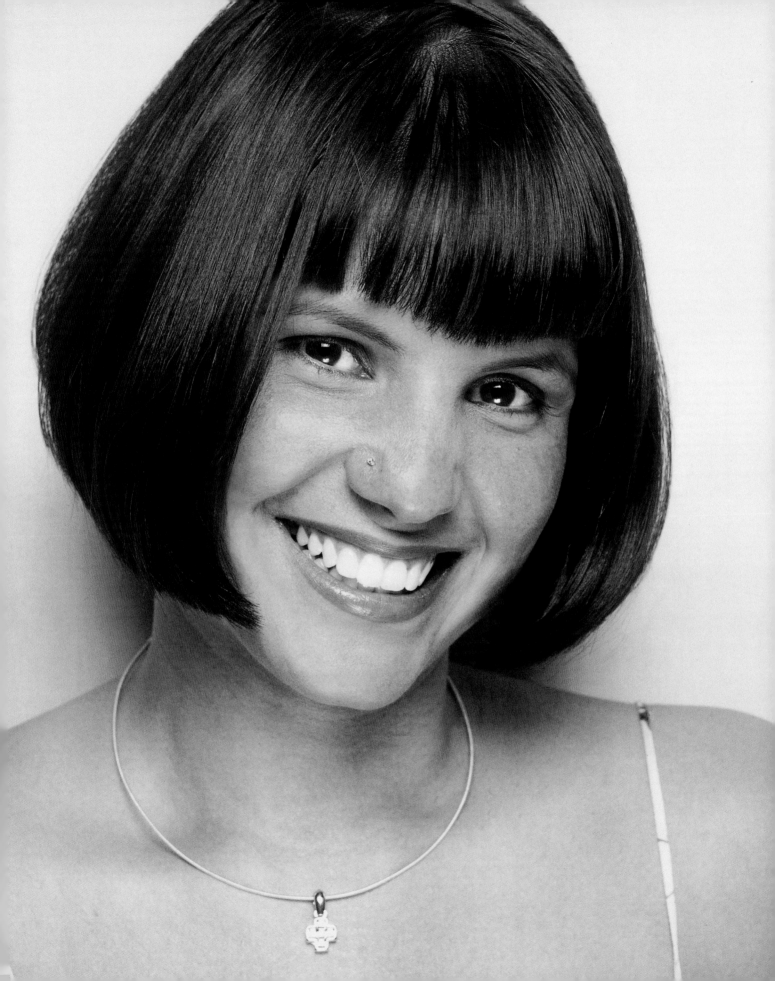

4. **Affirm** Yourself

AFFIRMATIONS ARE DECLARATIVE, POWERFUL, POSITIVE STATEMENTS that help achieve the state of mind necessary to bring about positive changes in your life. Timidity, shyness, indecisiveness, or a general *que será, será* attitude have no place in affirmations. Affirmations should be inspiring, galvanizing avowals that propel you toward feeling great, which in turn helps you do great things. Be bold. Be daring. Be fearless. Be *brava*.

Affirmations should not begin with "I hope . . .," "I wish . . .," or "I want . . ." Such sentiments only leave you hoping, wishing, and wanting—not a very fun place to be. Instead, affirmations should begin in the affirmative:

"I have . . ."

"Today I will . . ."

or, the most powerful affirmation of all,

"I am . . .," also expressed as, "*Yo soy . . .*"

You may feel as though you are being dishonest if you make declarations that are too far-fetched for where you are now. Say, for example, you are seriously in debt. Never create a statement that reflects your lack. In other words, don't say merely, "I will be out of debt," because that's all you will be: out of debt but most likely flat broke. Never limit yourself, sister. Reach higher. Do you really just want to be out of debt, or do you want a life that fosters enough abundance that money is no longer a worry and you can provide for yourself and your *seres queridos*?

You may be so in debt that creating a statement like "I have abundant wealth" seems ridiculous and laughable. This brings out another point when it comes to affirmations: Never say something you don't believe. A way to get around this, especially when you are feeling really down, is to devise an affirmation that is also an expression of thanks for what will happen. For example, "I thank God (or *la Virgen*, or the universe, or whomever) for bringing to me many opportunities to get out of debt and increase my abundance." When this happens, your affirmation becomes a prayer and an act of thanks all at once— a powerful combination.

5. Create Your Own
Sacred Space

FOR MANY OF US, WHILE GROWING UP A HOUSEHOLD ALTAR WAS A commonplace thing. It may have been elaborate, with large statues, flowers, candles, and burning incense. It could have been a plain white *vela* with a cross nearby. Or it may not have been an altar per se but simply a crucifix above the bed or an image of the Virgin somewhere in the home. Whatever we called it, whatever it was, the effect was the same: these objects and images were visual nods to a power greater than ourselves.

Latinos are well known for their home altars. *Curanderas* often set up ornate altars that enable them to help their clients heal. Altars are acts of faith made manifest, a part of our cultural inheritance from the women who shaped us. They are also beautiful tools to facilitate the presence of *ese algo* in our lives and in our minds. Altars are *ese algo* expressed in a physical form.

Perhaps you don't believe in God or have no particular faith. You still probably recognize the need to have a space that is your own.

The altars we suggest you create for yourself are not bound by adherence to a set of religious beliefs, since many faiths have different rules regarding what is and is not appropriate in that regard. This is more an altar about personal expression and the creation of a physical space that helps you to feel your best and, more important, to think in a positive, clear manner.

The most crucial function an altar serves, you will find after you've made your own, is in providing a space to give thanks, find stillness, and open your mind. Creating this space should be a fun and highly personal act, a way of expressing a side of yourself with objects you find beautiful, peaceful, funny, inspiring, or provocative. Don't worry about finding the "right" elements. When you decide to make an altar, the appropriate elements will cross your path.

Some ideas to help you get started:

Santitos

For those who come from a religious background and believe in the power of saints, looking for the right *santo* to reside in the altar is very important. While your selection will likely be driven by the message a particular saint holds for you, deciding how he or she will be represented is also key. Perhaps you have chosen *La Guadalupe*, the patron saint of Mexico. Thousands upon thousands of renderings have been done of her, and while they all have similar identifying characteristics, you should think about how you would like her to be physically present in your altar. You might choose a wood carving that is simple and clearly depicts her brown skin, or a printed cloth you can affix to the wall behind the altar. Or a tiny statuette might appeal to you more. Exercise your options.

Milagros

Common in Latin America, *milagritos* or *milagros* are usually tiny metal images

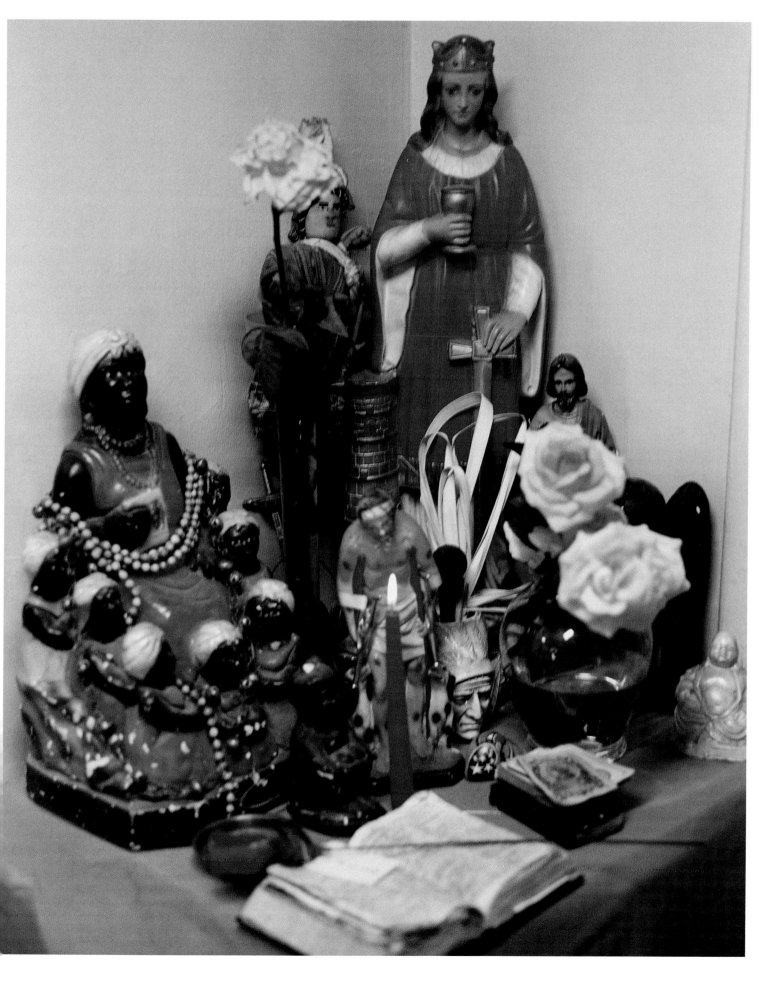

that look like charms. *Milagros* represent either a request for a miracle or a miracle granted. You will often find them at church altars around an image of the saint where the petition was made. They come in a wide variety of images, but there are a few common ones: a woman or man praying, an eye, the sacred heart, and an arm or a foot. The images are meant to evoke in some way the nature of the prayer answered or the supplication being made.

When deciding on an image, think beyond what the item itself depicts. A sacred heart, for example, could mean finding your heart's desire or your true avocation. A foot could represent the steps you are taking in choosing or creating your own *camino* in life.

You can even make your own *milagro*. The usefulness of *milagros* is that they symbolize exactly what it is you are expecting to bring forth in your life. Visual representations help you stay focused in your prayers and meditations and serve as reminders of what is truly important. When used to represent prayers that are answered, *milagros* serve as a thank-you gesture to God or to your higher power, as well as proof of the blessings you have in your life.

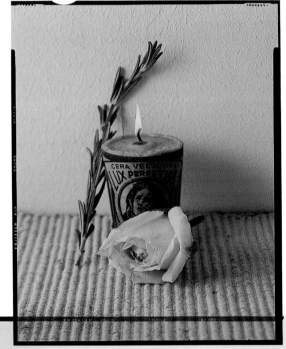

Velas

Purchase a seven-day candle, which comes in glass, or utilize aspects of aromatherapy by getting one of the scented candles that are so popular now. Certain fragrances are believed to be therapeutic. Lavender and chamomile, for instance, are noted for their relaxing properties and can help you reach a more meditative, de-stressed state.

Fresh flowers

Fresh flowers always lend an element of beauty and tranquillity to any room. Flowers also give a dash of color to brighten up a special place. Other components of nature, such as water, stones, and shells, have the same effect. It can be difficult, depending on your lifestyle and where you live, to maintain a steady stream of fresh flowers. If that's the case, you may want to consider a potted flower or forced bulb that lasts longer. Orchids, irises, and marigolds are lovely and last weeks at a time.

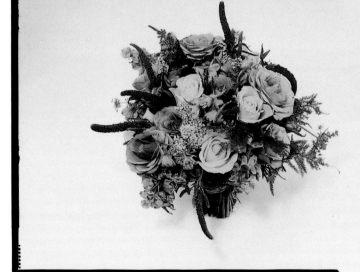

Incense

Some people dislike incense, while others consider it a necessity in building ambience.

So use it at your own discretion. Perhaps the greatest benefit of incense is that it lingers in the air even after it's finished burning, extending the aura it helped to create. An alternative to incense, if you really can't stand the smoke, are oils that release fragrance into the air when warmed.

Objects from your ancestors

Photographs of loved ones who have passed on—or even one of their personal articles, like a pipe or wallet—are profoundly affecting on an altar. Objects that represent these people keep alive the qualities they brought into your life, be it wisdom, unconditional love, knowledge, or inspiration.

Personal objects

Images or objects that represent things you would like to bring into your life function in a manner similar to *milagros*. They are the visual reminders of where you are going and what you would like to accomplish. Coins can represent abundance; candies can represent sweetness; a tassle from a graduation cap can represent the degree or certificate you will one day receive.

Collage

Making a collage for yourself is another way to evoke the life you have the potential to lead. Go multimedia: Don't just use magazines or newspapers; use sequins, crayons, photos, feathers, stones—anything you can possibly glue to a piece of paper. Some women create their collages on a box and place inside their written affirmations, prayers, and expressions of gratitude.

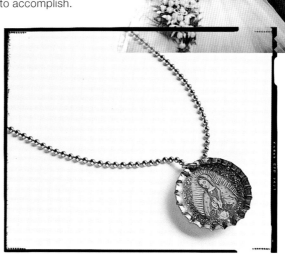

Photos from our ancestors (left, below) remind us that we are a part of something greater than ourselves. Personal objects, like the bottlecap Virgin Mary shown below, can have a religious or strictly individual significance.

"For those of us who are indigenous-looking—who have dark hair and dark eyes—we should be proud of that look and what we represent. Our looks show what our heritage is. We have to celebrate indigenous beauty, which is absolutely classic! My mother was Spanish, my father's parents were indios, and so I look Indian and I am proud of my look."

—DOLORES HUERTA, UNION ACTIVIST

Agua **Bendita**

BAÑOS ARE ANOTHER PART OF OUR BEAUTY *HERENCIA*. FROM OUR indigenous and African ancestors, we have inherited the knowledge that sometimes the simple act of taking a bath, when paired with the right intention, can be a powerful healing tool. *Curanderas* believe that baths can be sacred, a means of using water not only to cleanse but to heal, to release negative emotions and energies that are no longer useful to us. Baths can also be preparatory: a way to begin a new goal, to start a day of prayer, to open ourselves to new possibilities and ideas. Baths can be drawn around certain elements you would like to bring into your life, or simply to promote relaxation after a hard day.

Enhanced baths require extra attention. Set the mood physically, with candles or incense or through the selection of oils or herbs to help release specific energies or emotions. Set the mood psychologically by having a clear intention for your bath. Do you wish primarily to relax? To attain clarity? To create love? Know what you want as you are going into it. As in the creation of an altar, a *baño* can follow strict spiritual guidelines or be fed by a mix of elements—candles, fragrances, colors for the water—that are meaningful to you. To get started, here are two baths that are simple to create:

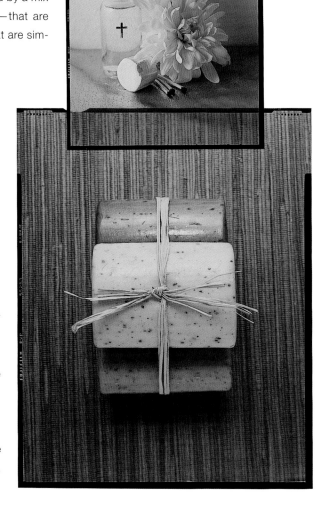

Relaxing bath

This *baño* releases tension and eases stress.

✔ Light candles throughout the bathroom. This is to create the proper *ambiente*. Make sure each is in a safe place, so you don't have to be distracted by them as you bathe.

✔ Tint the bathwater blue, to evoke the ocean. You can achieve this by adding bathwater colorants that do not leave stains—either on your bathtub or on your skin—and can be bought at drugstores.

✔ Add rose petals. Remove the petals from the flowers and scatter them on the surface of the water. Submerge yourself, surrounded by petals, and feel completely pampered.

✔ Mentally picture yourself releasing any tension or worries in your life. One exercise that is helpful is to picture yourself "giving over" your worries to the sea.

Love bath

This bath is not only for romantic love. In fact, it can be most powerful when used to facilitate love of yourself, your life, your family, or your friends.

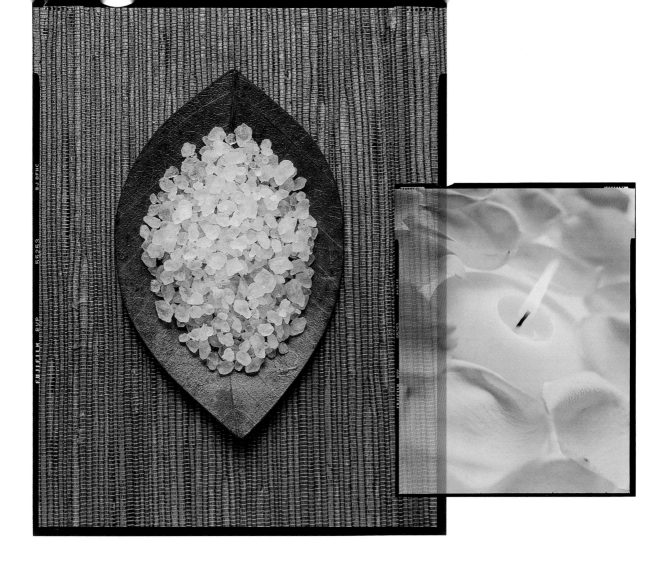

✔ Light pink candles throughout the bathroom.

✔ Add drops of rose oil to the bathwater.

✔ Tint the water a rose color.

✔ Add rose petals.

✔ As you take the bath, focus on your intent. If it is self-love you want to express, use the bath as a form of cleansing to forgive yourself for past mistakes and to release guilt. If it is a relationship you are seeking to create in your life, think about the person, as well as the type of relationship you are intending to develop.

Essential oils and herbal baths

These baths use oils, herbs, and properties of aromatherapy to help facilitate or evoke certain emotions.

- **Chamomile** (oil or dried)—calms and relaxes the nervous system.
- **Jasmine** (oil)—very feminine, puts you in touch with your inner beauty.
- **Lavender** (oil)—calms emotions, can help to facilitate deep sleep.
- **Rose** (oil)—promotes love of self and others.
- **Rosemary** (dried)—stimulates the body and activates mental and emotional clarity.

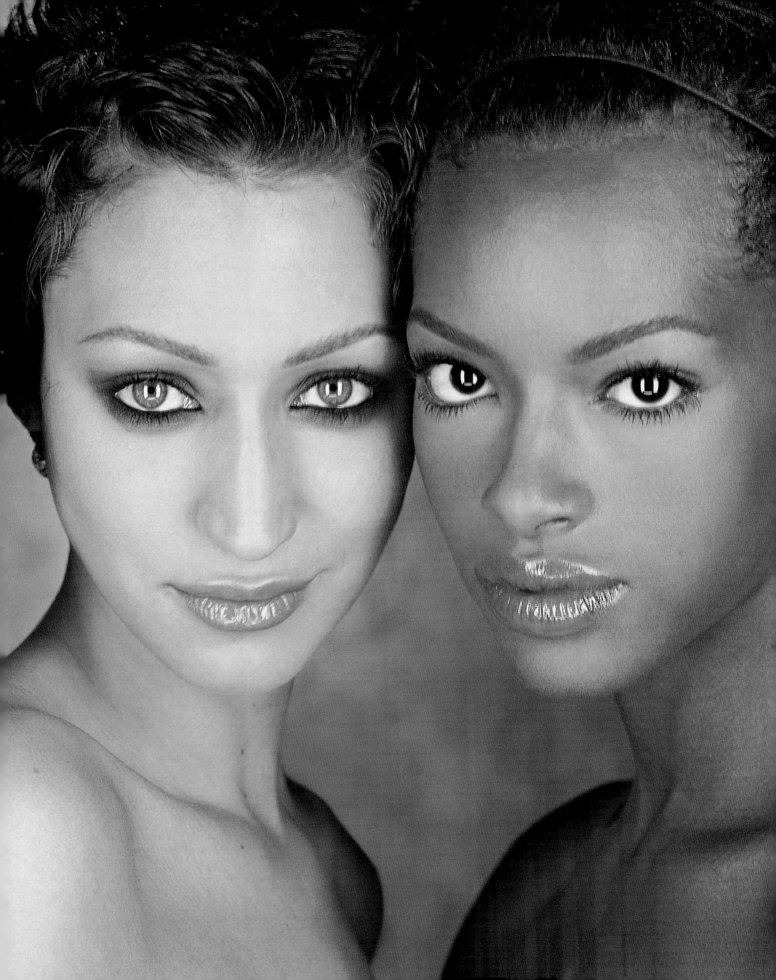

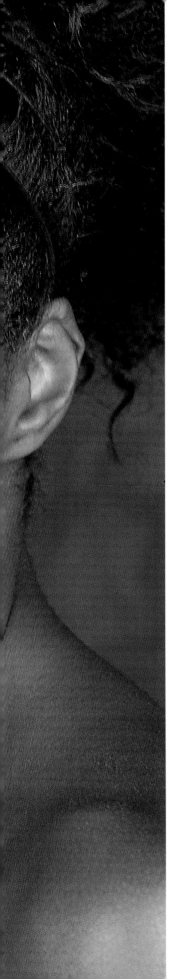

About Base:
Base, Powder, and Concealer

REMEMBER YOUR EARLY ATTEMPTS AT FINDING A FOUNDA-tion color that suited you? You went to the makeup counter ready to explore and to spend, and walked away feeling as if the only base colors cosmetics companies made were myriad variations on the same three tones: pink, pinker, and pinkest.

Meanwhile, you may have felt intimidated by those *hermanas* who, dissatisfied with what was out there, took it upon themselves to become mini-makeup experts, mixing their own foundation shades by combining different colors from different brands, all in a search for that perfect shade of honey or *café con leche* or *trigo*.

Here's the good news: Many makeup companies are finally waking up to the fact that most women—not just Latinas—have yellow tones in their skin. More important, they are beginning to appreciate that Hispanic women know and love cosmetics, and that we are not going to be satisfied with colors that don't work. But these days we find ourselves in a new predicament: With so many choices and so many different terms being thrown around, we may get overwhelmed and stick to a quick pat from our trusty powder compacts, the color we found in the ninth grade and have been buying ever since.

Not everyone needs foundation, and this is probably the most important lesson. Even if you wear foundation regularly, you may not need it every day because your skin is not the same every day. Some days you need more, some days less. As your monthly cycle comes, your body and skin changes, and having the right foundation, powder, and concealer helps to smooth and even out these variations. Whether you wear all three on a daily basis or only occasionally, the key is to find a color and formula that matches and enhances your skin color, not one that masks it.

Even a Latina with beautiful skin will benefit from having a foundation ideally suited to her face. Let's face it, you can't always be your usual flawless self. So instead of worrying about the imperfections, just grab your bottle of foundation, even out the tones, and get on with your day.

Another important lesson: Even if you do choose to use all of the elements, it's not necessary to use all three all over. Spot application, which we will explain later, allows you to take advantage of the benefits of makeup while letting your natural beauty shine through.

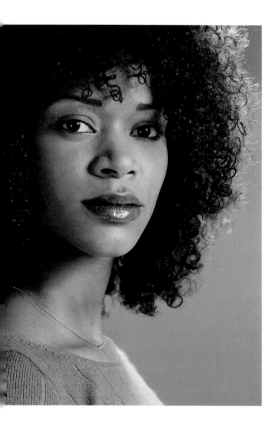

Some Latinas mistakenly use foundation to change their skin color, either going too light or too dark. Base, concealer, and powder should enhance your natural skin tone and camouflage any flaws, not change the skin color entirely.

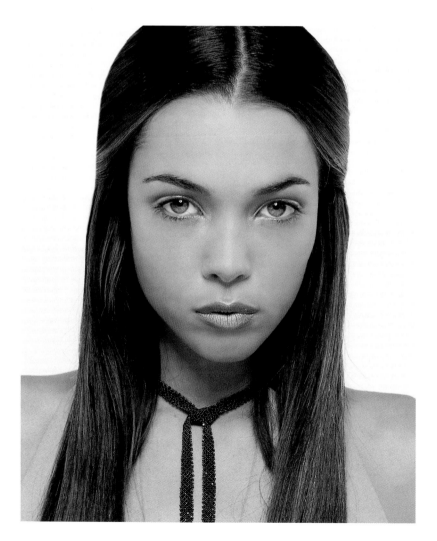

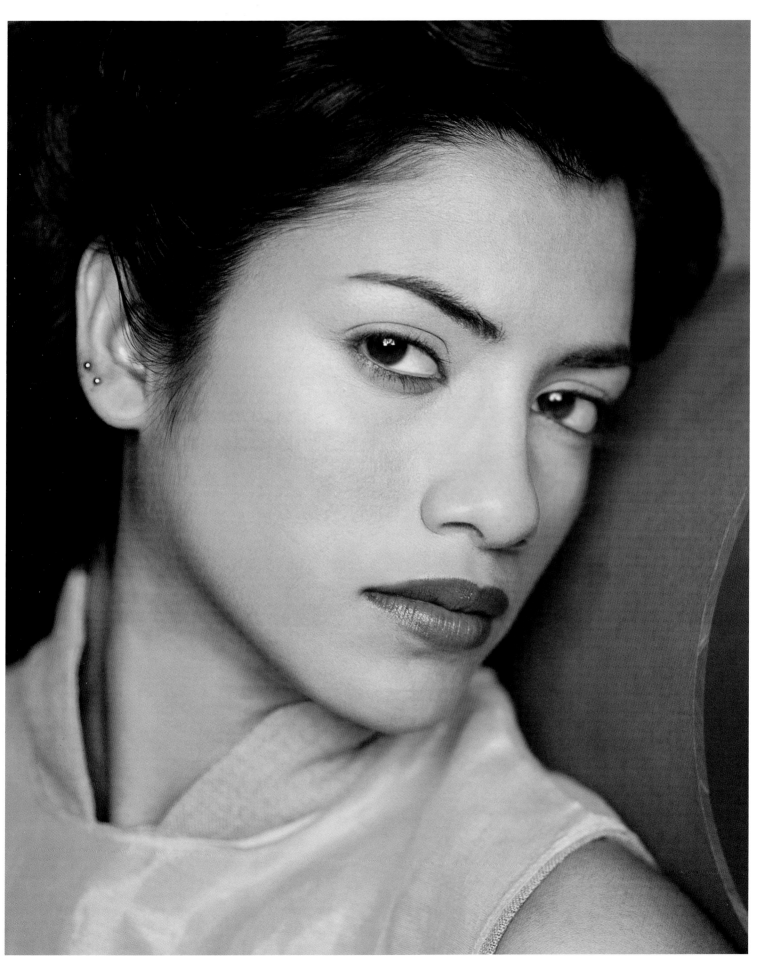

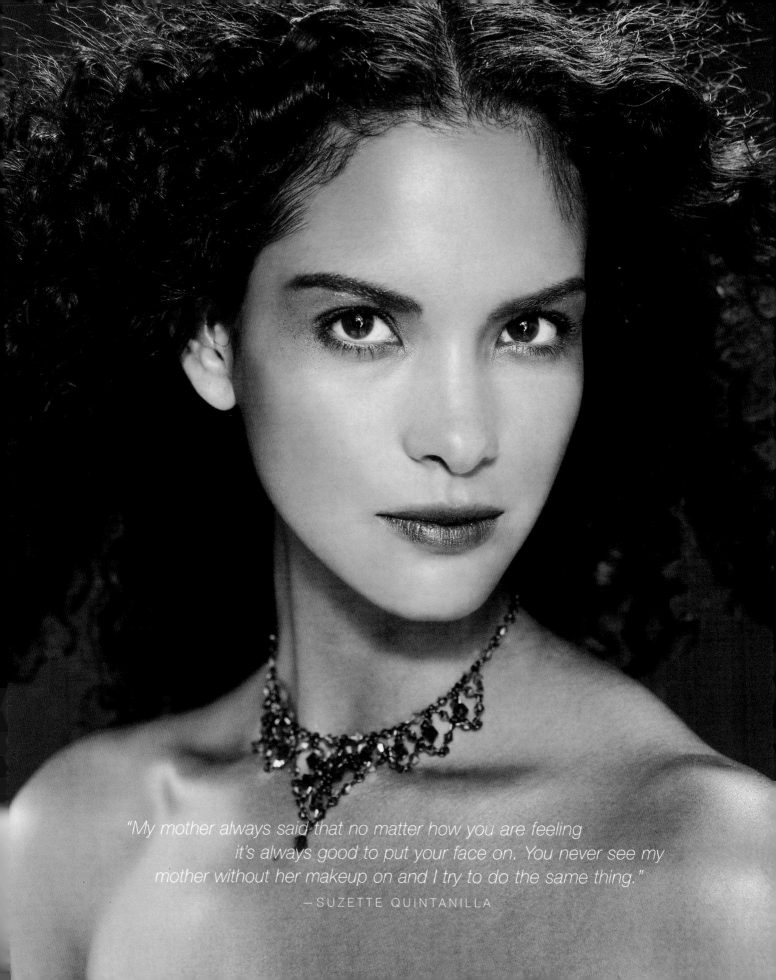

"My mother always said that no matter how you are feeling it's always good to put your face on. You never see my mother without her makeup on and I try to do the same thing."
— SUZETTE QUINTANILLA

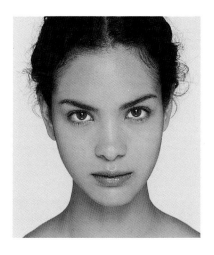 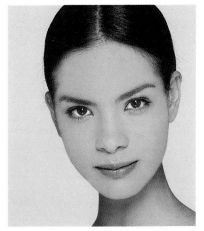 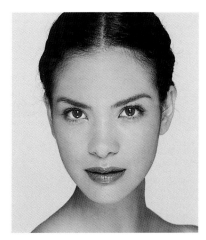

Who, when, and why

When it comes to foundation, women tend to fall into two categories—those who use none and those who use too much. These two camps can learn a lot from each other, because the best place to be on this continuum is the middle ground.

Where is the middle ground? Quite simply, it changes according to your needs. If you are going to a business presentation and you want to look fresh, energized, and focused throughout the day, the best solution is to apply the foundation—and concealer and powder—with a slightly heavier hand than normal. The makeup will wear well as the day goes on, and, more important, you will be able to focus on the presentation, not on whether your face is starting to shine. On the other hand, if you are going to spend the day outside playing softball with your *cariño*, a light application is all that's needed. Whatever the occasion, though, pretty much everyone can benefit from a little foundation.

The winning formula

Finding the right color may have been the primary concern back in the days when the only options for women were liquid or pancake makeup. But now, with advances in formulas and skin care, women can select foundations that do a number of jobs beyond just evening out the skin. The foundation you choose should be influenced as much by your lifestyle as by your skin tone.

There are certain things to keep in mind:

• **Your skin type:** Whether you're dry or oily or in-between, you have particular needs.

• **Your skin texture:** If you have smooth skin with fairly small pores, your options are a lot wider than those of someone with acne scars, hyperpigmentation, or large pores.

• **Your expectations:** Do you have only three seconds to apply foundation and want that application to be almost foolproof? Do you have more time and the patience to blend well? Do you want to correct blotchiness, or do you simply want a wash of color?

The different levels of coverage in foundations create three distinct looks. From left to right: Sheer coverage, best used on nearly flawless skin, gives just a light wash of color; skip the powder to keep a dewy "no-makeup" feel to the skin. Medium-coverage foundation, like the kind most liquid foundations give, achieves a more polished, even skin tone. Full-coverage foundations, like the one pictured far right, tend to be matte and impart a heavier, traditional "made-up" look.

Foundation **Forms**

Stick

Stick foundation offers a more finished look and, when applied correctly, can also double as a concealer. Best for normal-to-dry skin, it is also a good option for women who want more coverage from their makeup—either to even out blotchiness and correct uneven skin tones or to ensure that the coverage lasts well into the day. Sticks are becoming very popular for their versatility and compact form. They do require a bit more blending than their equally versatile cream-to-powder counterparts, but overall, they are easy to use.

Stick: Versatile and easy to use.

Liquid

Liquids are what we all grew up with. The beauty of liquids is that they come in a myriad of formulas, which means you are likely to find one that matches your skin type. You can also control the amount of coverage it gives. If you want a sheer look, mix it with moisturizer or sunscreen. If you want more coverage, simply apply more. This versatility also means that liquid can be used on a variety of skin textures.

In general, when applied straight from the bottle, liquids offer more coverage than sheer formulas but less than sticks or cream-to-powder formulas. In terms of expectations, if quick, flawless application is what you are looking for, liquid may not always be the best route. We've all seen the battle scars left by hurried application: unblended, cakey streaks along the neck or cheek. Liquids require time.

Liquid: Medium coverage that blends well.

Sheer

Sheer foundations and tinted moisturizers provide the least amount of opacity and coverage, allowing for quick blending. These are excellent for women with great skin who just want an all-over evening-out of their skin tone. Sheer formulas should be avoided like the plague, however, if your skin tends to be oily, blotchy, or has an uneven texture. A sheer foundation is useless for correcting these problems.

When sheer foundation was first introduced, a lot of cosmetics companies offered them in a smaller color range than they did other foundations. That tendency is changing. Sheer formulas can also accommodate a larger range of skin tones, since they allow more of the woman's skin tone to show through. It is still necessary to select a shade as close to your skin tone as possible, though;

Sheer: For a hint of color and complete blendability.

foundation just a shade off can make the skin look strange. In any case, due to the popularity of sheer foundations and tinted moisturizers, many companies, especially in the mass-market segment, are rapidly expanding color choices.

Cream-to-powder: The solution for on-the-go coverage.

Cream-to-powder

For a woman who has no time and wants a matte finish with a high amount of coverage, cream-to-powder formulas are an excellent option. These formulas are kinder to oily skin than their stick counterparts because the powder helps cut down excess shine. Cream-to-powder foundations with a slight sheen to them, a new alternative, provide a lot of coverage without the matte quality. These should be chosen carefully, however, since, as anyone with oily skin knows, you don't always need help in getting that "glow." But women with normal-to-dry skin will love the moister formulations and how easily they tend to glide on. Anyone whose skin texture demands more coverage (large pores, blotchiness, or acne scars) should stick with mattes.

Foundation **Formulas**

Matte

Matte foundations can come in virtually every form—stick, cream-to-powder, liquid—with the exception of sheer. What a matte foundation does is essentially take away any shine. In more technical terms, matte foundations absorb light, while non-matte or iridescent formulas reflect light. Generally, matte foundations are excellent for anyone who has oily skin and wants a lot of coverage, or who wants their foundation formula to last throughout the day.

Matte: Oil-free formulas are best at cutting shine.

Iridescent

Iridescent: For those who want to glow.

Iridescent foundations are relatively new. These generally sheerer formulas, which contain light-reflecting particles that give the skin a nice glow, must be blended well and don't have the staying power of traditional foundations. Iridescent foundation is an excellent choice for older women with very small pores but should be avoided by women with oily skin, no matter how much the person at the department store touts it as the "new thing." At the most, an oily skinned person can spot-apply it to areas like the cheeks or around the eyes. But there is no reason to buy a new foundation for this purpose when other tools like highlighters or an all-over shimmery powder can create the same effect.

Skin-Treatment
Foundations

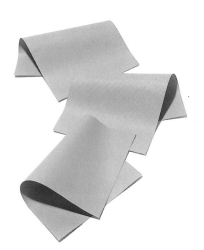

SKIN-TREATMENT FOUNDATIONS TEND TO COME IN LIQUID OR CREAM-to powder forms. In addition to offering the basic service of a foundation, they provide additional benefits to your skin, most popularly—and most usefully—sunscreen protection. If you can find a foundation with a broad-spectrum sun-protection factor (SPF) that suits your skin type, texture, and skin color, by all means buy it. If you have oily skin, make sure the formula won't add to the overabundance of oil your own skin produces. You might prefer to apply an oil-free sunscreen, skip the moisturizer, and then apply your foundation. Darker-skinned Latinas should check what ingredient is providing the sun-screen protection. If it is titanium dioxide, make sure it is micronized titanium dioxide, or you can end up with an ashy look to your skin.

Pore-clearing (also called skin-clearing) formulas contain acne-fighting ingredients like salicylic acid or exfoliants, such as alpha or beta hydroxy acids. These can be effective for women who have mild acne, but bear in mind: If you are also using a stronger acne medicine that contains the same ingredients, the skin may become dry and quite sensitive. Second, the coverage might not be to your liking—either too sheer or too opaque. Use your best judgment and your own skin's response when trying these new foundations. Certainly, anyone who uses a strong prescription acne medication should avoid these foundations. But since these medications cause sun sensitivity, sun protection must be a priority; buy a separate dermatologist-recommended sunscreen and apply it before using foundation.

Oil-absorbing foundations can be a godsend to women with particularly oily skin. Some makeup artists maintain that any oil-free foundation, when followed with an application of good loose powder, is enough. Try a few formulas and decide for yourself. You might find the elimination of that extra step of applying powder to be the biggest advantage of oil-absorbing foundations.

Maestro minuto

NEW YORK CITY-BASED MAKEUP ARTIST AND photographer Ezequiel de la Rosa swears by one little-known, low-cost beauty product he says really works: blotting papers. These little sheets come in envelopes or booklets and can be purchased at drugstores and upscale department stores. Whatever the brand, the effect is the same: They absorb excess oil on the surface of your skin, matting out the face while keeping makeup intact. You can keep the sheets handy in your purse for touch-ups throughout the day. Some varieties leave a layer of fine, light-colored powder on the skin to further absorb oil. Be wary of these powdered sheets; if the shade of powder doesn't match your skin, they can leave you looking like you just stuck your nose in a bag of flour.

Selecting the **Right Shade**

AGAIN, THIS IS WHAT MOST AGGRAVATES AND ANNOYS LATINAS WHEN it comes to the beauty industry. So much attention has been paid to finding the right foundation color that now, depending on the company you buy it from, you get numerous "theories" about undertones and all manner of color-matching techniques created in an effort to make makeup buying "easier." Many of us just end up feeling confused.

The bottom line is this: Latina skin tones generally come in different shades of brown. For most of us, this means we need to look for foundations with yellow or golden tones, as opposed to pinks. Even *las más güeritas*—those who turn pink instead of brown under the sun—can benefit from a yellow-based foundation, since it will minimize any redness that appears from irritation, blemishes, or blushing.

If you are looking for a new foundation and want to get a sense of how much yellow is in the formula before applying it to your face, the best way to judge is through comparison. Take an obviously yellow-toned foundation—even if it doesn't match your skin tone—and apply it on the back of your hand. (Remember, you are only attempting to judge the amount of yellow used in the formula, not to select a shade to apply on your face.) This foundation is what you will use as your control shade. Then, apply a streak of the color you are considering on the same hand near the area you applied the first yellow foundation. By looking at the two shades together on your skin, you will be able to tell immediately which formula has more yellow in it. Try applying a third streak from another line of base. The differences will become even more obvious.

Once you have settled on a line or group of colors that have enough yellow for your satisfaction, it's time to pick your shade. The best place to test foundation is to apply it where you are going to wear it: on your face. Not your neck; not your arm; not the back of your hand: *la cara*, and that's it. To really select a color effectively, do it on a sunny day, take a good-size hand held mirror with you, and step outside and see for yourself how the base matches. To speed up the process, apply three dots of color to the area beginning at the hollow of your cheek and going down to the edge of the jawline. One dot should be the shade you think matches you best. The next should be one shade lighter, and the third should be one shade darker. If you are on either extreme of the color spectrum (very dark or light) or of the range of shades the makeup line makes, apply a second shade anyway. The practice of comparing colors will help you gauge more effectively if your first choice is right for you. If none of the colors you have applied look right or make you feel confident about the choice, move on to another line of foundations.

If you still can't find exactly the right shade or are torn between two, you'll have to use your skin texture as a guide. If you have very even, clear skin, you can afford to go with the lighter shade. For those with the occasional blemish, the darker shade is the better bet. The reason: Light colors accentuate, while darker colors warm up the face, helping to camouflage imperfections.

Remember that foundation is not completely opaque; it should blend with the skin, not cover it. Think of it as your skin, but better. Foundation is the starting point for everything else you will apply to the face, and you may end up wearing it every day. So it's worth the time and money spent to get it right.

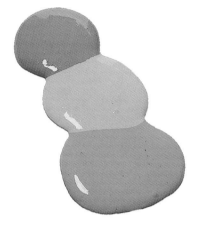

Un Tip Rapidito

Comparing colors on the back of your hand, for all makeup, is a wonderful way to learn to better appreciate the nuances in shades. What looks like the same neutral lip liner from three different makeup companies can, when applied to your skin, reveal a wide variation of pink, brown, or orange. You may also stumble upon an inexpensive color that is the exact replica of one from a far more expensive cosmetics line—another benefit of comparing colors on the back of your hand. Obviously, what looks a certain way on your hand will look different from the way it looks on your face. This technique is simply a way to be aware of the difference each item has from another.

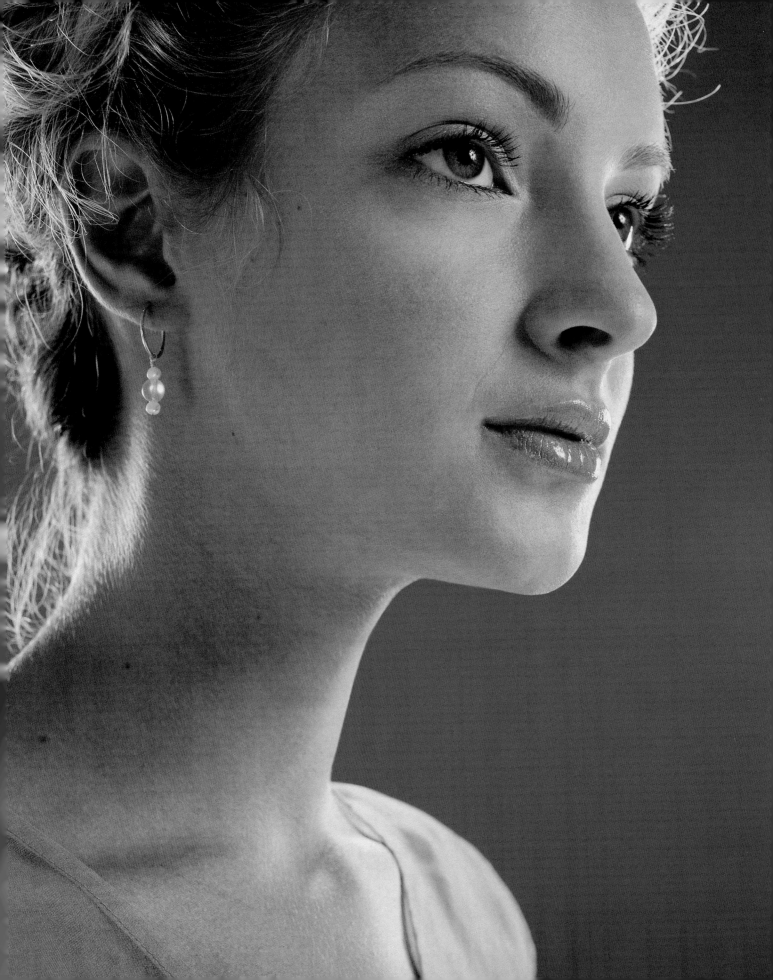

Tips for fair-skinned Latinas

For fair-skinned women, the normal irritants that affect most people's skin become magnified. Any redness, irritation, blemishes—even hyperpigmentation or *manchas*—become showcased. Because of this, it is especially important to steer clear of pink-tone foundations and stay well within the yellow-to-golden-tone-foundation range.

Tips for dark-skinned Latinas

Many foundations—and even many powders—are made with a white pigmented powder called titanium dioxide. Titanium dioxide has recently resurged in popularity because it has been found to be one of the only ingredients to offer broad-range protection from both UVA and UVB rays of the sun. Any products with this ingredient give an ashy cast to the skin when applied to women with darker complexions. In fact, even light-skinned women who apply sun-protection factor (SPF)-formula sunscreen with titanium dioxide can end up looking like a geisha girl on the beach. Read the label carefully to make sure that there is no titanium dioxide in the formula or, if there is, that it is micronized titanium dioxide. Micronizing grinds the powder so finely that there is no ashiness. This is also important to remember when it comes to selecting a daily SPF-15 sunscreen.

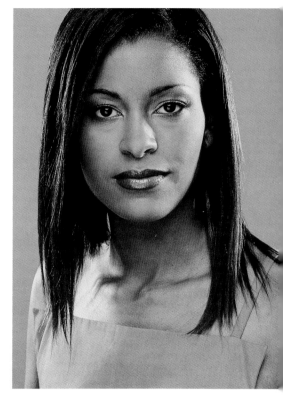

These Latinas (opposite, above) got their foundation right; they wear shades that match their skin tone and bring out the beauty of their complexion.

Foundation for the summer

Despite all of the warnings regarding skin cancer (we will talk more about that later) a lot of *hermanas* still insist on tanning during the summer months. Even for those of us who do use sunblock religiously, the fact is we tend to brown very easily, even with a daily dose of SPF 15. This means that the foundation we use during the winter months doesn't look right as the days get longer and the skin gets darker. Since your skin color isn't the same year-round, your foundation should change with it. The best solution is to have "winter" and "summer" foundations you can mix during any transition periods. Use the same selection technique when it comes to color, but also take into account any climate changes and subsequent skin changes you may go through. An oil-absorbing formula might be better for the hot summer months, even for a woman who has normal-to-dry skin in the wintertime.

Application tips

Some women prefer to apply their makeup with sponges, others with their fingers. Ultimately, it's a matter of choice. If you have oily skin, sponges may be the better way to go, since the oils that are naturally present on your hands won't get mixed in the makeup you apply to your face. Sponges also allow for more precise application in the crevices of the nose. Since sponges do absorb some of the foundation, you may feel as though you are applying more foundation when you use your fingers. This can be controlled by simply being aware of how much you use. Some makeup artists use foundation brushes, as you will note in Chapter 10 ("Celebrity *Secretos*"). Brushes do help with a smooth application and are excellent for blending a mix of colors.

Polvo Primer

POWDER HAS MANY FUNCTIONS. IT CAN BE USED TO:

• **Set foundation.**

• **Even out skin discoloration.**

• **Minimize shine.**

• **Prepare eyes, lips, and lashes for further makeup application.**

Loose powder

Loose powder is most commonly used to set your own foundation after application, followed by an extra application on the T-zone (the nose, chin, and forehead) for oily skin.

Techniques for applying loose powder vary. A large powder puff or a sponge provides an even surface for application. A fluffy powder brush doesn't apply the powder as evenly, but it has the advantage of preventing powder from caking on the skin. In order to ensure the smoothest application, tap the brush first to loosen excess powder. Using a flat, round makeup sponge instead of a puff or brush gives slightly more coverage. Some women can simply apply powder this way and be ready to go, skipping foundation altogether.

If your intent is to set your makeup, or if you have a tendency toward oily skin, then pressing the powder on with a puff or a sponge is the most effective method of application. To reap the greatest rewards, however, it is important to literally press the puff onto your skin in repeated motions, not press the powder on and then smudge it around the rest of your face. Think of it as spackling the powder onto your face.

Loose: Gives the best finish to set your makeup for the day.

The main areas you want to be sure to hit with powder are your nose and the area around it, your chin, forehead, and lightly around the eyes. Powder should be used with care when it comes to the eye area, however. Matte powder, in particular, when applied with a heavy hand, can accentuate fine lines around the eyes. The cheeks tend to be drier areas of the face and don't need as much, if any, powder.

Pressed: For touch-ups only.

Pressed

Most makeup artists recommend pressed powder as an on-the-go option, not to be used instead of loose powder. This is simply because loose powder has far superior setting qualities. Pressed powder was never meant to replace loose powder altogether; it was meant to be a convenient alternative. It's also important to note that some pressed powders have oilier formulations, so women with oily skin should probably choose oil-absorbing or oil-free pressed powder.

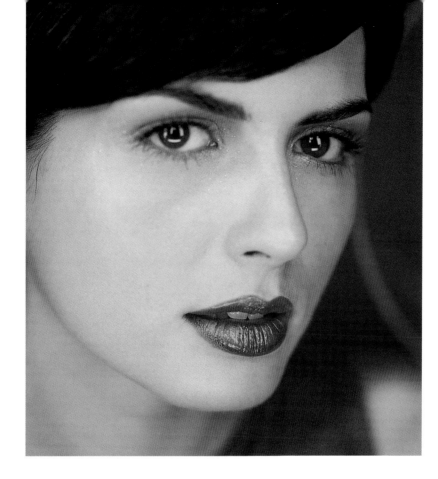

Powders were once used strictly to eliminate shine. Now the most popular formulas enhance radiance, as well.

Shimmery

Shimmery powders are similar to iridescent foundations in that they contain light-reflecting particles that give the complexion a dewy finish. Although people with oily skin should normally avoid iridescent foundations, shimmery powders can be a nice way of achieving the same glow without the oil.

Translucent

Translucent powder has less pigment in the formula than regular loose powder does. It sets the makeup and blots out shine without adding color. Women of all skin tones can use it, providing the powder contains no white pigment. White pigment will look ashy on darker skin tones.

Shimmery: Use sparingly, and strategically, wherever you want to gleam.

Un Tip Rapidito

Most of us have had this experience: We apply foundation, then dust on powder only to find that our face turns a nasty orange color. According to Miami-based makeup artist Fátima Olive, the moisture in a foundation can cause powder to "bloom," or pick up the moisture of the base and thus turn a darker color. To prevent this, either wait until the foundation dries completely or select a lighter color of loose powder.

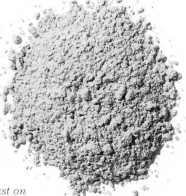

Translucent: The works-on-almost-everyone alternative.

Concealer **Weapons**

CONCEALERS ARE A WOMAN'S BEST FRIEND. IF MEN ONLY KNEW THE power wielded at the end of a sponge-tip applicator, there would be a concealer shortage that would leave many an informed *muchacha* exposed and irate. Unlike foundation, which some women consider a choice, almost everyone needs concealer at one time or another. Far more opaque than foundation, concealers provide the highest form of coverage for the skin. Even among concealers, there are different levels of opacity, and hence different formulas can be better suited to some needs than others.

The rule with concealer, though, is that you should only apply it where you need it. If the inner corner of your eye is where you have excessive darkness you would like to cover, apply concealer to that area only, not the entire under-eye area.

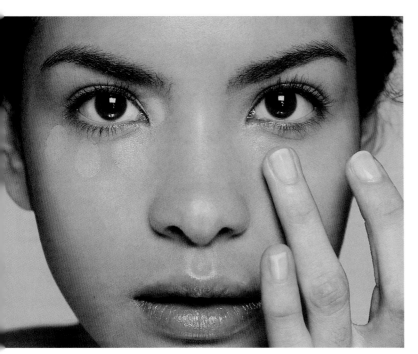

Eye-ay-ay

Eye concealer is a basic step in making up the eye (which we'll get into later), but even if you are only wearing mascara, applying some concealer can brighten up the whole area, making you look awake and refreshed. Yet the eye area, the most common place to use concealer, can also be the trickiest. The key here is to find the right formula. If you use a formula that is too moist it can cause slippage, ending up in the creases and fine lines around the eye and drawing attention to what you don't want people to see. A formula that is too dry is bad for the delicate skin around the eye and also magnifies fine lines. You will need to experiment to find which formula is best for you.

Place concealer where you need it. Around the eyes: Dab on lightly with ring finger. Below: Creamy concealers are better for the under-eye area, as they are easy to spread and blend without tugging the delicate skin.

The latest batch of concealers that are especially effective for the under-eye area contain light-reflecting ingredients. Oddly enough, a number of these formulas come in pink shades, which might generally cause Latinas to reject them immediately. Don't be so quick: These products really work. Formulated in a very smooth liquid that is easy to apply, the concealers don't actually camouflage as much as brighten the skin. This means one shade can be used on a wide variety of skin tones. Look for concealers described on the packaging as "brightening" or "illuminating."

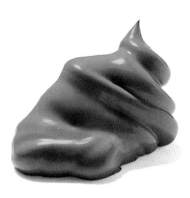

Blemish blenders

Covering a pimple is not the same as applying concealer to the under-eye area, or to any areas of your face, for that matter. In fact, if you have to cover up blemishes regularly—even if it is only one or two at a time—consider purchasing a different type of concealer for that purpose. While a concealer for other areas of the face, especially the eye area, can and should be more moisturizing, you need the exact opposite quality in order to conceal a blemish effectively. Some of the new long-wearing or transfer-resistant concealers are drier and extremely effective in this regard.

The second thing to remember is a concept we spoke of earlier: using light and dark tones to manipulate appearance. Remember, white reflects light, thereby magnifying; dark absorbs light, thereby minimizing. Most women choose a concealer that is a tad lighter than their skin tone, which is excellent for certain areas of the face, such as the eyes or around the nose. But a blemish is a raised bump on the skin. Clearly, in order to draw attention away from the raised area, it's better to choose a dark concealer over a light one. One very important point: Choose a concealer that is only a tad darker than your skin.

Sometimes the area around a blemish tends to be slightly oily, making it hard for the concealer to adhere to the skin. Counteract this by applying a light dusting of loose powder beforehand, helping the makeup to stay in place and wear well throughout the day.

When covering a blemish, a concealer brush can be very helpful, since it allows for more precise application than your finger. One common mistake women make is to cover up around a blemish instead of directly on top of it. Use the brush to apply concealer on top of the blemish and around it only if it is needed. For fair-skinned Latinas, whose blemishes tend to be accompanied by a lot of redness surrounding the pimple itself, apply concealer around, being sure to blend the concealer well into the surrounding unaffected area.

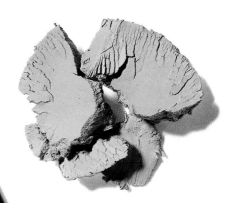

A thicker, more opaque concealer, applied with a special concealer brush, works better on blemishes.

Manchas and Freckles

MANCHAS, HYPERPIGMENTATED AREAS OF SKIN, ARE TRICKY TO cover up. If the spots are significantly darker than your skin, an opaque concealer is the best option.

When selecting a color, however, the mistake a lot of Latinas make is to select a color that is too light in an attempt to counterbalance the darkness of the *mancha*. This only results in an ashy-looking mess on your face. Choose a concealer that helps blend the darkness of the *mancha* with the lightness of the surrounding skin—in effect, a color darker than your skin but lighter than your *mancha*. This is a technique that requires time, patience, and practice.

The same goes for freckles. Most people now find freckles to be attractive, and many would even suggest forgoing trying to cover them altogether. If they concern you, choose a color that is slightly darker, not lighter, than your natural skin tone. This only works when your *pecas* are few and far between. Unlike with *manchas*, however, select a sheerer formula to cover up freckles; you might even consider simply sticking with foundation and skipping the concealer.

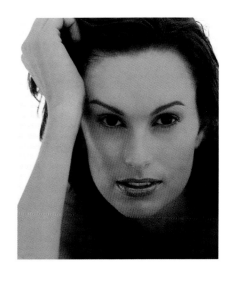

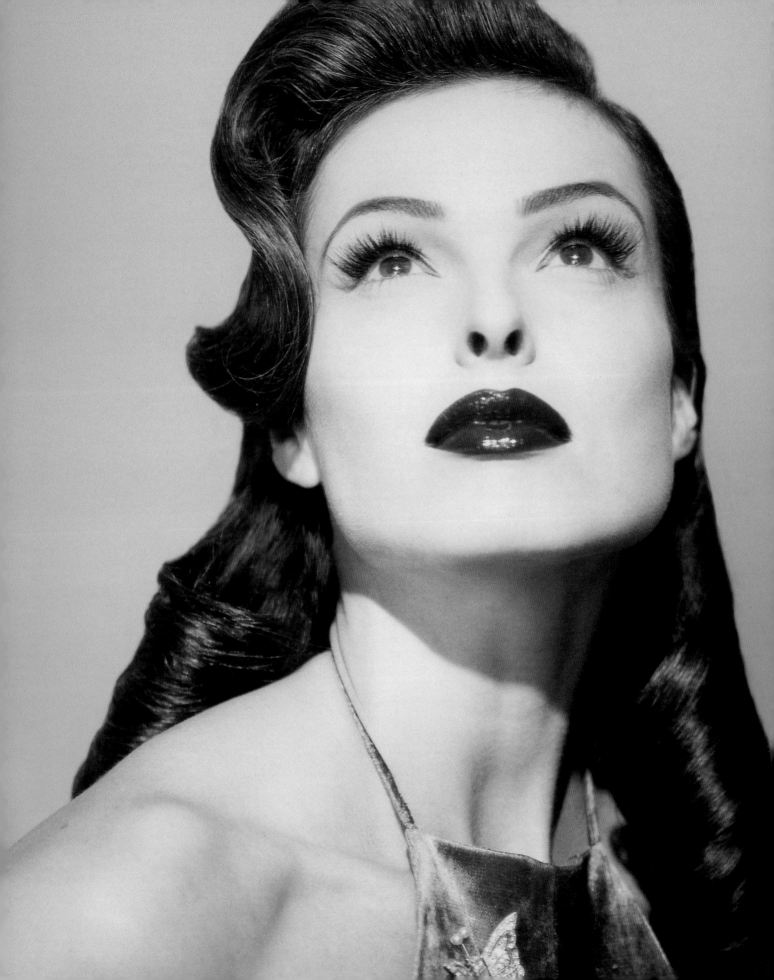

Blush & **Pout**

THERE ARE SOME LATINAS WHO MISTAKE THEIR BLUSH FOR war paint. Sporting streaks of purple on each side of their face, they look ready for battle when they step out the door. Other Latinas avoid rouge entirely, figuring they have enough color as is.

Depriving yourself of the benefits of blush is a mistake, since it can accentuate the beauty of brown skin, making it look healthy and glowing. The key is to understand what blush can do and to apply it in the right way.

Blush, depending on how you use it, can:

- Add color.
- Define bone structure.
- Emphasize certain parts of the face while de-emphasizing others.

Blush

ONE BIG MISTAKE WOMEN MAKE WITH BLUSH IS TO OVERUSE IT IN the fall, in an attempt to compensate for lack of color when we start to see our tans wear off. This technique usually fails and instead draws attention to the pallor. You also go wrong when you select colors that are too red or purple for your complexion. The third most common error when it comes to blush is in using a strong color, then proceeding to apply too little, so that by the end of the day almost no color is left on the face.

Blush, highlighter, and contour powder used together create a dramatic look like the sculpted, contoured face below.

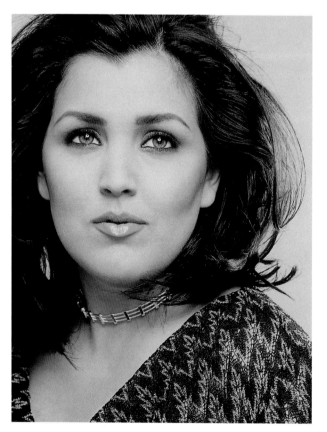

Selecting the right shade

Your goal should be to find the most neutral shade that will still add color to your face. For most women, and especially for everyday wear, you should select a color that makes you look healthy and goes with your skin tone and almost all the makeup colors you wear.

Notice how your skin looks after you have just worked out, or when you blush naturally. When blood rushes to the face, it registers on the skin as a shade of pink. It could be a deep pink, a light rose, or even an almost tanned, peachy color for those with browner skin tones, but the base is always pink.

The amount of blush you use, rather than the color, is what will be subject to change on a day-to-day basis. Depending on the amount of color you have on other areas of your face, you may need less or more blush. If you are wearing a strong lip color, you can turn down the blush that day, since the color element of your makeup is already there. If you are wearing a wash of beige on your eyes and a neutral lip, you will need more blush to still have a nice amount of color on your face. Even the colors worn next to your face can affect how much blush you should apply; a bright pink scarf wrapped around your neck brings enough color to the face that your blush that day can be less strong.

More sophisticated makeup users occasionally change their blush shade along with the rest of their makeup color

*"My inspiration comes from my family and also from my faith.
I am Catholic, and I'm constantly asking to be inspired. I'm constantly
in prayer for everything that I do. I'm a big believer
that we're all vessels for something much greater."*
—TATYANA ALI

palette. Rosy cheeks, when paired with some pink lip gloss and pastel eye shadow, for example, make for a whole different look that warrants the change from the subdued neutral you may usually wear. Oranges, purples, and even deep reds are trend-oriented looks you can experiment with but are difficult to use every day.

Selecting the right formula

As with foundation, the type of blush that will work best for you depends on your skin type and texture. A third factor to take into account is your skill level. If you are comfortable with make-up, you are ready to experiment. If you are not willing to spend an exorbitant amount of time learning a new technique, stick to what you know.

Powder

Powder is the easiest form to use. It is also suited to more skin textures, since powder doesn't draw attention to flaky skin the way liquids or gels can. Powder is also the best option for people with oily skin or big pores. Powder blush should be applied to the face after you have applied your foundation and set it with loose powder. If you are wearing powder blush but not foundation, apply the blush after you have applied your sunscreen or moisturizer. Powder adheres better to a slightly moist surface. Applying it straight to dry skin may result in your losing the color faster as the day wears on.

Cream or cream-to-powder

These types of blushes are excellent for women with skin that is normal to dry or dry but not flaky. Oily skinned Latinas should avoid cream blush unless the formulas state explicitly that they are oil-free. If you have large pores, you should also avoid this type of blush. The benefit of using a cream is that, when applied well, it looks very natural and it has long wearability. Creams or cream-to-powder blushes should be applied after moisturizing or after foundation but before applying loose powder. Powder will tone down the color slightly, so you can afford to apply a little bit of extra color.

Liquid

Liquid blushes are good at imparting a light flush to the face, but they require a higher skill level in terms of application technique. The formulas dry on the skin quickly, requiring you to blend rapidly after application. Liquid blush works by literally staining the skin, so you must have a smooth, even skin texture to begin with before using it. Liquids, like gels, are also harder to find. So when you do find a makeup company that makes these formulas, chances are the color range will be a bit limited. Liquid blush should be applied after moisturizer or after foundation, if you are wearing base.

The type of blush selected affects the final look. Powder blushes (above) are more traditional, while reflective particles in some cream blush formulas (right) give an added glimmer along with the color.

Un Tip **Rapidito**

Powder blush has to be applied with a brush—don't even think about using a sponge—because the application must be even and cover a fairly large section of the face. If you invest in a good blush brush, you can afford to skimp on the price of blush itself. Selecting a good blush brush isn't hard: Use your face size as the best guide. Small women don't need a huge blush brush, for example. Still, the brushes included with most blushes are generally too small for any face size.

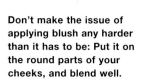

Gel

Gel should only be used by women with highly refined skin, as it has a tendency to fall into pores. If you have large pores or pores that clog easily, a gel blush will draw attention to the problem. Gel blush should be applied after moisturizer or foundation.

Applying the blush

The issue of where to apply blush is simple: Brush it onto the apples or fleshy parts of your cheeks that protrude when you smile widely. Women get confused when they start to use blush to contour or use bronzers to heighten tans. But blush is simple: Keep it on the *chachetes*.

Don't make the issue of applying blush any harder than it has to be: Put it on the round parts of your cheeks, and blend well.

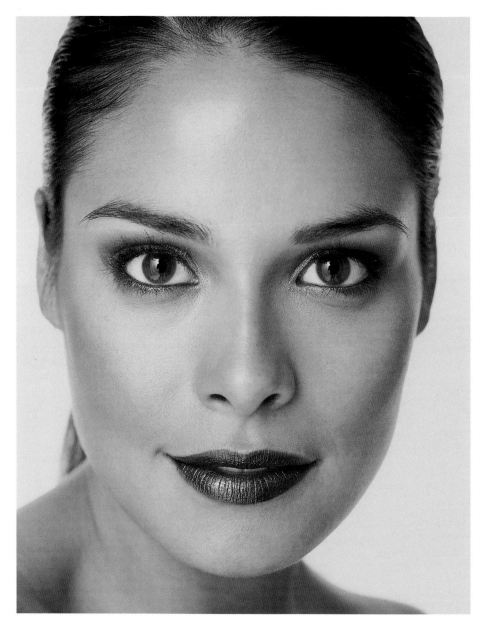

Bronzers

THE BIGGEST GAFFE with bronzer is to use it all over the face. The objective of a bronzer is to mimic the effects of the sun. When your face gets tan, the sun doesn't hit it evenly; some parts get more brown more quickly. Also, in applying bronzer to the entire face, you miss out on an excellent benefit: the depth and "sculpting" effect it can have.

Selecting the right formula

Powders

As is true with blush, powders are the easiest form of bronzer to work with. They also suit the widest variety of skin types and are the clear best choice for Latinas with oily skin. If you use a powder bronzer, purchase an extra brush for application. Using the same brush for both blush and bronzer will only muddy up both colors. The other option is to clean your brush thoroughly after each use—but who has time for that?

Sticks

Stick bronzers are popular because most have a slight sheen to them, imparting a dewy, fresh look to the skin. The rule here is the same with shimmery foundation: It's best for people with normal-to-dry skin.

Applying the bronzer

Put it where the sun would shine: the cheeks, nose, chin, and forehead. Some women use bronzer and skip the blush, but if you add your regular blush lightly, it amplifies the golden-rosy tone the bronzer is creating. If you already have a deep tan, you may need to switch to a darker blush as well.

Bronzers should give a warm wash of color that mimics the way the sun hits your face. Used correctly and sparingly, the effect is natural and fresh, deepening already brown and beautiful skin or lending a warm glow to fairer-skinned Latinas.

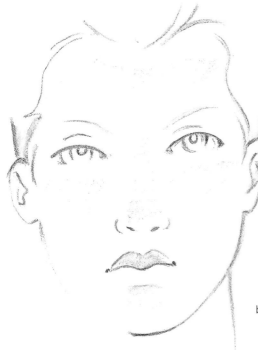

Creating **Illusions**

CREATING CONTOURS ON THE FACE IS A LOT LIKE PAINTING. YOU USE light and dark colors to define and create more dimension. This technique never looks good in broad daylight. Any woman who thinks that by contouring her face she can get rid of her *papada* is fooling herself. But properly done, contouring can create a dramatically new look for the evening or for a photograph. Do not try this for everyday wear or for being in daylight.

To contour effectively, you need two separate colors: a darker hue to accentuate hollows or receding areas of the face and a lighter color to bring out features that look better played up. Start with you own skin tone. Find a contour powder that is no more than three shades darker and a highlighter powder no more than three shades lighter. Anything too stark will be difficult to blend. Powder is the most effective method; it's far easier to blend than foundation and easier to correct if you have made a mistake. You can use your bronzer to contour the areas you want to recede, but since bronzers sometimes have shimmer in the formula, it may be best to buy a separate matte dark contour powder. It is also a good idea to have two separate brushes. Use a smaller one for applying the light powder, allowing for precise application, and a slightly larger one for the darker color.

Begin by applying the lighter color first. This will prevent you from getting too heavy-handed (and streaky or muddy-looking) with the dark colors. And always remember to blend, blend, blend. A lot of women want to use contouring around the jawline to slim down their faces or minimize a double chin. Attempting to do this is very tricky, as the jawline is one of the hardest places to blend effectively. Make sure to have someone else there who can look at you and judge whether the makeup is seamlessly blended.

Contouring is being used by women less and less, since it is so hard to do well. Also, going to a cosmetics counter and asking to look at their selection of contour powders will get you either a blank stare from the salesperson or a tour of their assortment of blushes. If you decide to do contouring, stay away from using blushes. Opt for pressed powders in darker or lighter skin tones instead.

Never use your blush to try and create defined contours in the face. Rely on highlighting and contouring products to give shape, reserving blush for color.

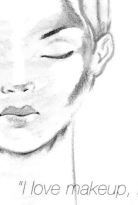

"I love makeup, but when I am not working I prefer to look natural. If I'm just going out I wear mascara, pink color on my cheeks, and gloss on my lips."
—VALERIA MAZZA

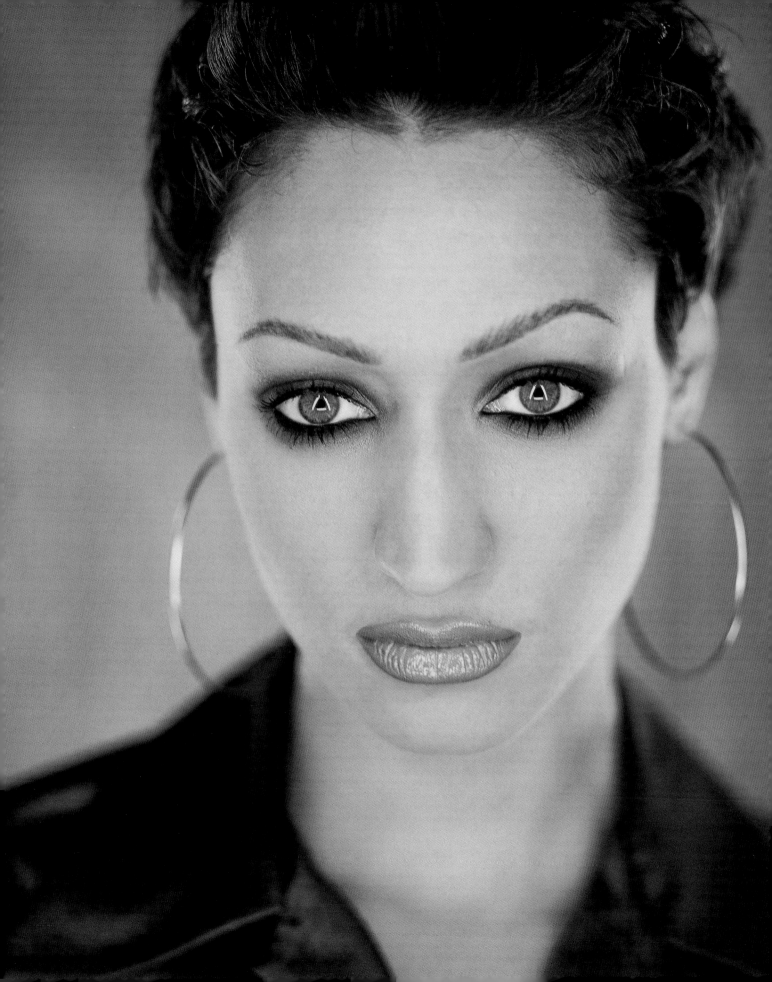

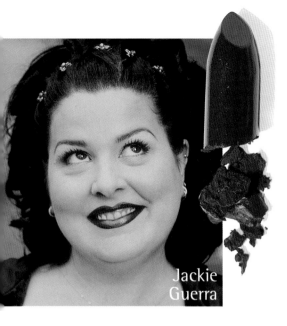

Jackie Guerra

◄matte

The type: No shine, little moisture, high opacity. Needs to be applied with brush for precision.
The look: Very glamorous. Very strong.

creamy►

The type: More moisture than matte and easier to apply. Gives the vivid color of matte without the flatness or dryness.
The look: Feminine, classic, and sumptuous.

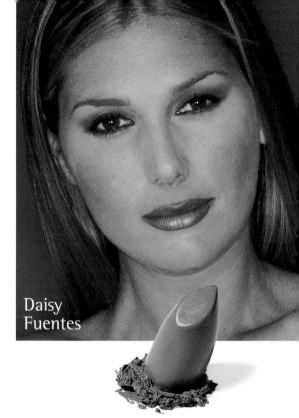

Daisy Fuentes

Labio Lessons

A WOMAN WHO DOESN'T EXPERIMENT WITH A WIDE VARIETY OF COLORS, TEXTURES, AND TECHNIQUES when it comes to her lips is really missing out. Even the most minimal makeup routine should include a lip color.

Guide your lipstick choices in terms of formulas and the effect you are trying to achieve, rather than just by color. With such a great array of shades to choose from, don't let old rules dictate your look. And don't worry about selecting the "right" red or the "perfect" pink, because the rule for lipstick and color choices is simple: The more you play with different colors, the more aware you will be of what looks best on you. Experimenting with different tones will also make you more attentive to the overall effect a lip color has on the rest of your makeup. As we mentioned before, with strong red lips, you will be able to tone down the blush you apply. The bottom line: Lips are for fun, *m'ija*.

Here's a primer on differences in formulas and suggestions for which look each is best suited for.

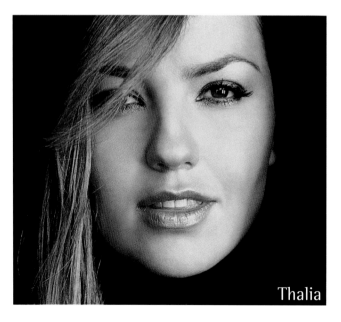

Thalia

◄frosty

The type: Has the consistency and staying power of cream, but the reflective particles add depth to the lip.
The look: Voluptuous, sexy.

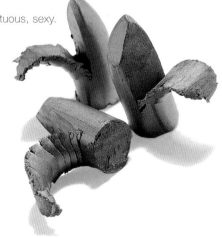

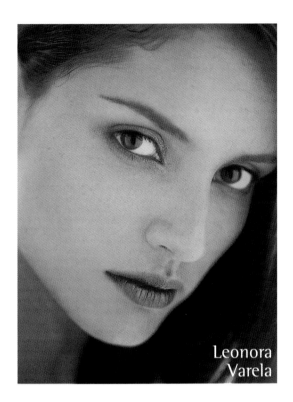

Leonora
Varela

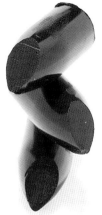

◀ sheer

The type: Less pigment than creamy or matte. Lets you see the skin through the lip color.
The look: Clean, simple, and sensuous.

Christina
Aguilera

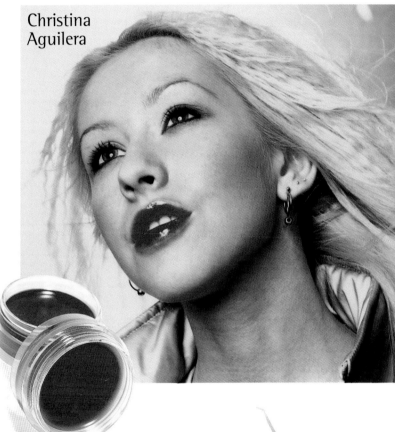

gloss ▶

The type: High shine. Varies from clear to outrageous, bold color.
The look: Youthful, fresh, and fun.

Tatyana
Ali

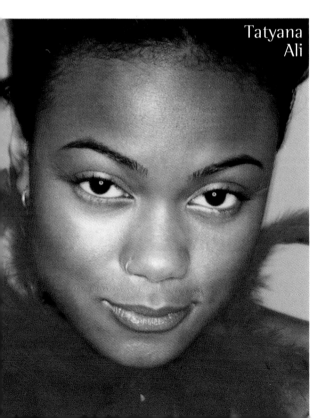

◀ shimmer

The type: Like a gloss, but with reflective, glistening particles in the formula.
The look: Disco diva, a more sophisticated look than gloss.

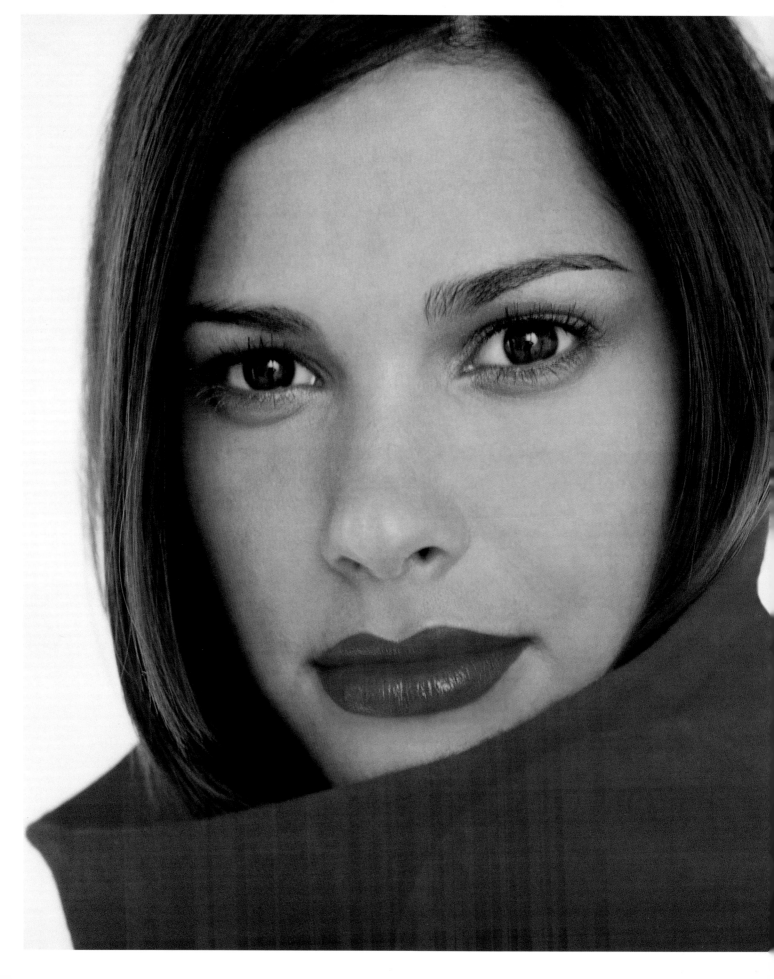

Lip liner 101

SOME LATINAS WE KNOW FORGO LIPSTICK ALTOGETHER AND just stay with lip liner. These women realize what a friend lip liner can be; used correctly, it adds definition to the lip line, extends the wearability of lip color, and even lends a hint of dimension and fullness to the lips. Lip liners come in varied forms, mostly pencil, but the size of the pencils and the creaminess varies from brand to brand. It's ultimately a question of personal choice. In any case, there is one inalienable truth when it comes to lip liners: They are useless unless they are sharpened. It's staggering how many women will drop $15-$20 on a good lip liner, yet not pay the extra $5 to get a high-quality sharpener. Quality does make a difference. Bad sharpeners can actually cause the wood in the pencil to splinter. There are better ways to get the illusion of bee-stung lips without poking them with a splinter of wood from your lip-liner pencil.

All lip-liner pencils are not created equal. If, as you draw the pencil across your lips, your lip goes with it, the formula is far too dry. The pencil should glide smoothly across the lip surface, leaving a fairly strong pigment.

Application technique using lip liner and lip color

Here is the easiest way to apply lip liner:

Start at the perimeter of your lip line and, using light, feathery strokes, bleed the color inward toward the center of your lips. This allows you to blend the color as you apply it. If you are following the liner with an application of sheer lipstick, don't overapply the lip liner, as it will defeat the purpose of the sheer lip color.

Applying the liner in one solid stroke is fine for those already adept at lip liner application. But for novices, it can be easy to distort the line of the lip accidentally. Also, keep your mouth slightly open as you apply, since this keeps the lips closest to their natural shape.

The dark lip liner/light lipstick "issue"

THE IDEA BEHIND THIS IS A GOOD ONE: THE GRADUAL TRANSITION FROM DARK TO LIGHT IS supposed to give the appearance of full, pouty lips. *La palabra clave* here, though, is "gradual"—if you don't blend, you simply end up with a dark purple or brown line encasing the lips and a light glaze of color on the inside. If anything, not blending can actually make the lips look smaller because you are encasing your lips with a thin (or thick, as the case may be) line. Too much contrast can kill this look.

If you are trying to alter the shape of your lips—we'll tell you how later—still follow your lips' natural shape with lip liner for the preliminary application. Changing the shape will require you to build on the shape you already have.

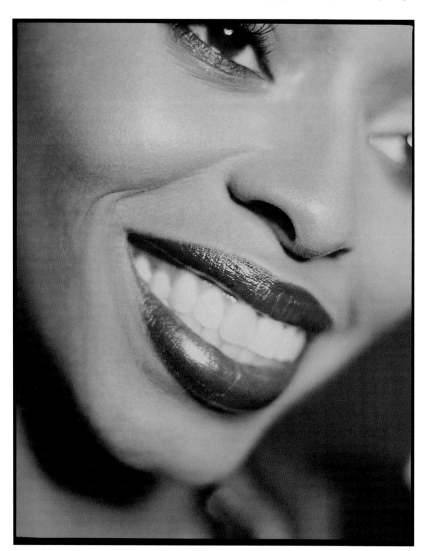

Once you have drawn the basic shape of your lips, step away from the mirror and take a look at yourself from a distance. Taking a step back is a good thing to do at numerous points in the process of applying makeup, since most people are not going to look at you while standing three inches from your face. Stepping back helps you keep a sense of balance and a lighter (or heavier, when needed) hand in terms of the overall impact you are creating.

When you are satisfied with the shape you have outlined, you are ready for the lipstick. Many women wonder if applying lipstick with a brush as opposed to straight from the tube is really such a big deal. If you want your color to last, and you don't want half your lipstick to come off with the first cup of *café con leche* you drink at the office in the morning,

Some women have skin tones on the lips that are different from those on their face. To even everything out, apply a light layer of foundation over an application of lip balm, creating a smooth, even canvas to paint up a pair of fabulous, sensual *labios*.

Did you know? Latinas make up 11 percent of the U.S. female population, but account for 17 percent of lip liner used nationwide.

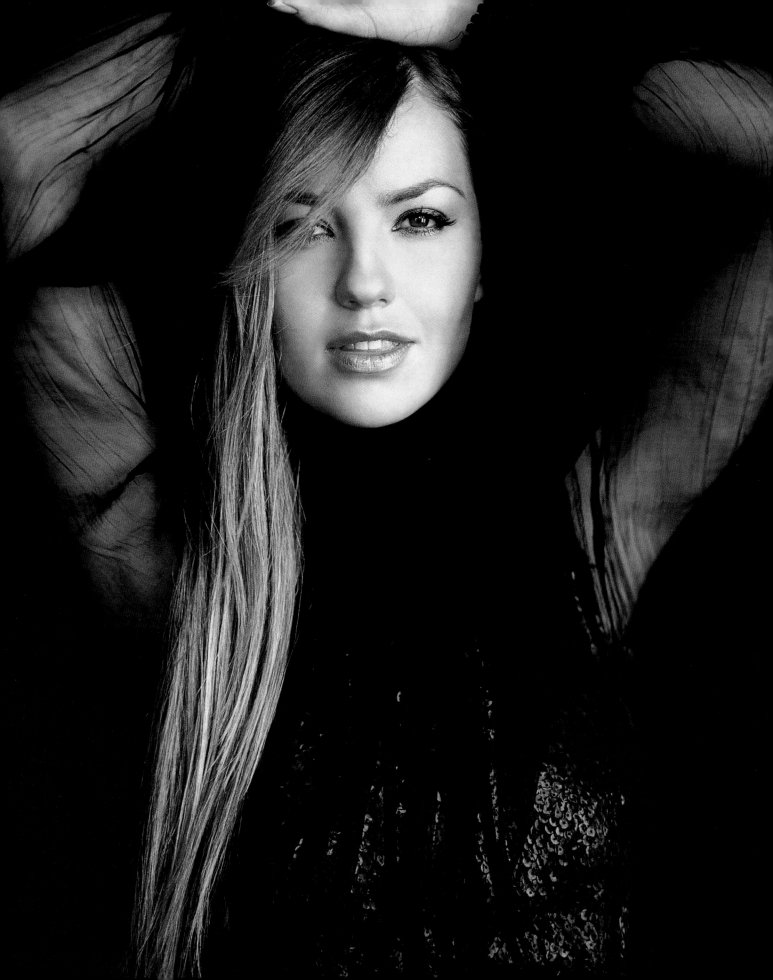

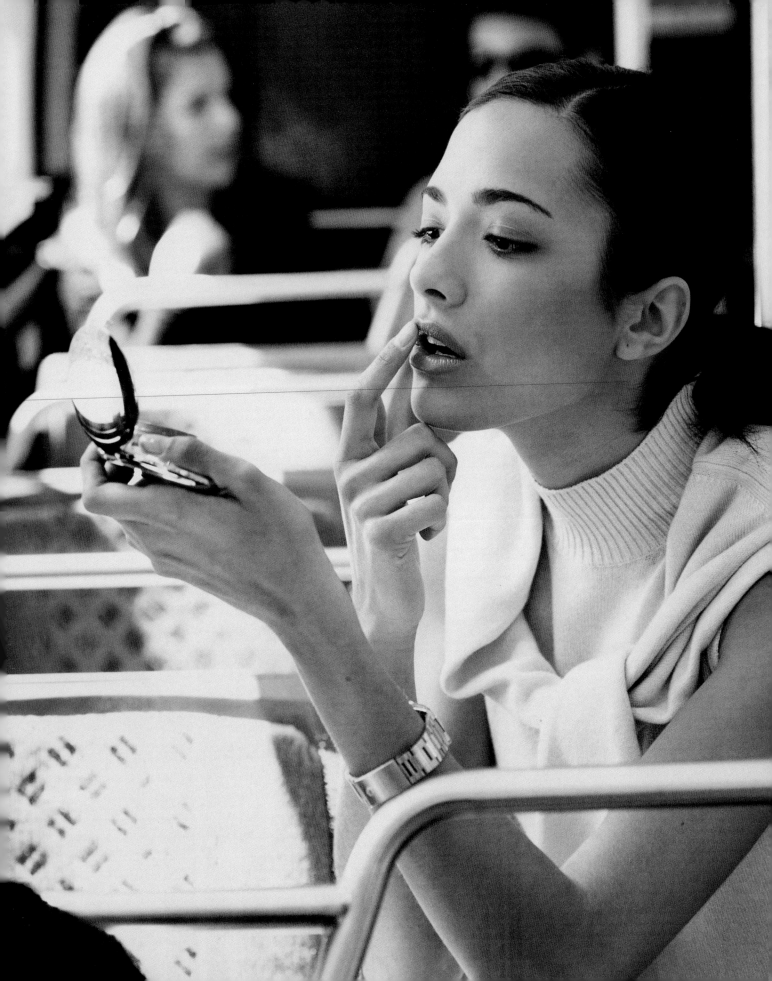

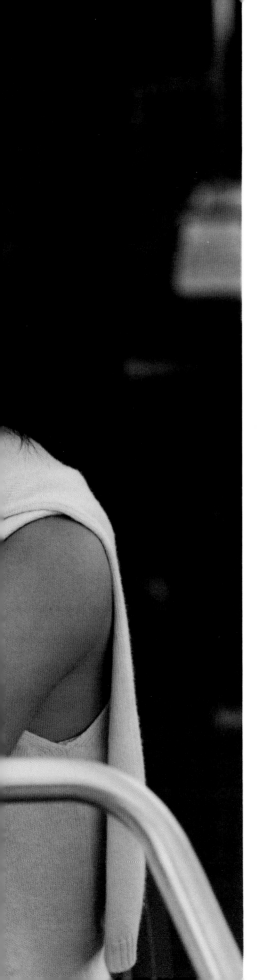

brush application is much more effective. You'll use less product, but more of it adheres to the lips, and the pigment is more evenly distributed. Applying lipstick straight from the tube leaves more pigment on the lips, and often too much—the excess can bleed into any fine lines around the lips. Blotting the lips with a tissue, a technique to remove excess lipstick from the lips, is an unnecessary step when applying color with the brush. A brush allows for more precise application, which is important when you are creating vampy, matte lips à la Rita Hayworth or using a complicated lipstick application technique, like changing the shape of your lips or creating the illusion of pouty, full *labios*.

Creating **Illusions**

Making fuller lips

The sort of highlighting you use to create curves and bone structure on the face can also work on the lips. Apply a light, matte lip color to the center of the lips, which draws light and creates the illusion of fullness. Apply your final lipstick color on top. If your final lip color is sheer you have to be sure it blends well, but this technique can be used with darker sheer lip colors and creamy lip colors of any shade. The old trick of applying gloss to the center of the bottom lip lasts as long your lip gloss—which is to say, not very long. If you want the illusion to last, stick to our technique.

Altering lip shape

Begin by drawing your natural lip line with the lip liner. This creates the base from which you can alter the shape. After you have drawn in your lip shape, draw the areas you are seeking to reshape. Whether you are extending your lip line to make the lips appear larger or you are doing it to add more symmetry to a pair of lopsided lips, it's good to select lip color carefully. Stick to neutrals and light colors, since a dark red or bright purple calls enough attention to your lips as it is. Bear in mind that as with facial contouring, changing the lip shape rarely looks natural. It's best to stick to your natural lip shape for everyday wear.

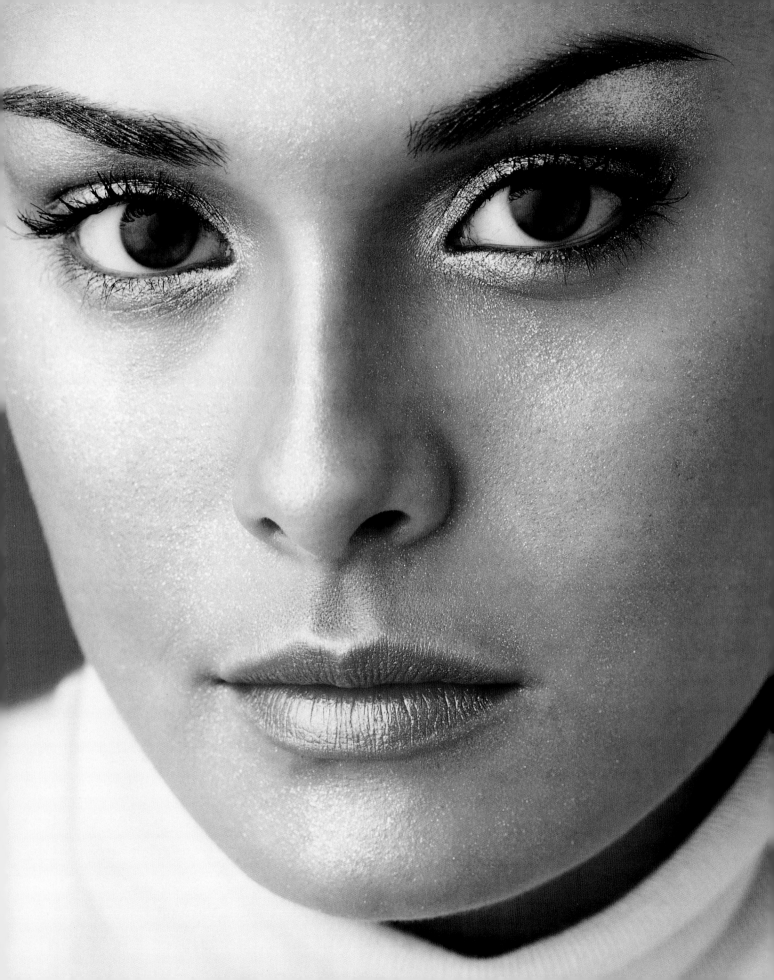

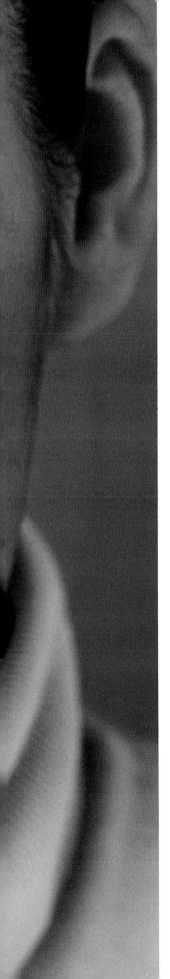

Luminous *Ojos*

IT'S TRUE: THE EYES ARE THE MIRRORS OF THE SOUL, revealing emotion and thought. They also reveal lack of sleep, an excess of fun the night before, and the urgent need for a *siesta*. You want people to be attracted to the shiny, sparkling orbs that are your *ojos*, not the scary, unwelcoming bags that are your *ojeras*. Most *muchachas* realize this and as a result have become adept at applying concealers and waving mascara wands over their lashes, as if that is enough to grant the wish for glowing, amazing eyes. What a lot of *hermanas* miss is that, with a little extra effort, the eyes and eyebrows can dramatically change our appearance.

Being able to adapt a look is particularly important for us. As we know, Latinas come in all shades and colors. An eye-shadow color that appears to be of medium intensity and pigment will look very light on a darker-skinned Latina. Often a sister will see a beautiful eye makeup look on a Caucasian or African American model, and instead of thinking, "How can I make that work on me?" will simply say, "That looks beautiful on her, but I could never pull it off." This mindset is limiting and untrue. Learning the right application technique and knowing your eyes frees you to explore the possibilities and to bring out the beauty of *tus ojos*. Before we even go into makeup application for the eyes, however, a brief word on the eyebrows.

Serious *Cejas* Smarts

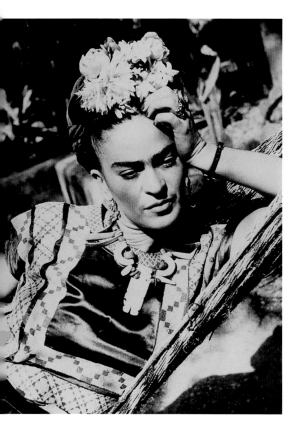

Frida Kahlo's disregard for popular standards of beauty and her embracing of her own unique *belleza* meant that she followed what she thought was beautiful.

The trick for grooming *cejas* that grow down: Comb the *pelitos* down (their natural growth pattern). Trim any hairs that extend below the brow line. Allowing the brow hairs to lay in the direction they grow prevents them from looking unruly.

A LOT OF BEAUTY BOOKS GIVE A SIDEBAR ON EYEBROWS AFTER THEY have taught you how to apply eye makeup. This is a mistake. Eyebrows are the frames of the eyes. They should complement, not compete with, this main feature of your face. Give yourself a great pair of brows, curled eyelashes, mascara, and some undereye concealer, and you are ready to go. A good brow can do as much for your eyes as an eye lift—and it's only a fraction of the cost.

The goal when you are attempting to do your eyebrows, or going someplace to get them done, is to make them look better than they do naturally, not to dramatically change the entire shape of the brow. But if a night out calls for a glamorous look, the brow can be the detail that takes you from a plain *Juana* to a beauty *reina*.

As Frida Kahlo showed, many of us have a lot of brow to contend with. Frida wore her unibrow loud and proud, defying traditional notions of beauty and facial hair for women. Frida was special: She developed a look so unique to her that no one could imagine her without her dramatic eyebrows, or her moustache, for that matter. She not only kept her eyebrow hair exactly where nature put it, she made her *pelitos* part of her artwork, rendering each individual hair in her self-portraits. Most modern Latinas, however, don't feel comfortable wearing brows the way Frida did. Although her own self-assuredness in her femininity and beauty sets a wonderful example of not trying to change who you are, we don't think you have to be embarrassed about experimenting with eyebrow wax or a pair of tweezers.

First, the basics about eyebrow know-how. In general, tweezing or waxing is the eyebrow hair-removal method of choice. Tweezing is good for shaping and to do fine detail work, like accentuating your natural arch. Waxing is a better option for women who have never had their brows done before, or who have substantial amounts of eyebrow hair to remove.

An eyebrow wax simply involves applying warm wax on areas where excess hair needs to be removed. A muslin or cotton strip of cloth is placed

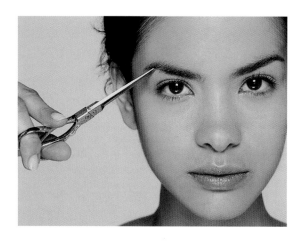

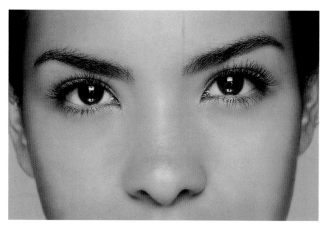

over the wax. With one swift tug, the cloth strip is removed, taking with it the hairs that were covered by the wax. Possible side effects include redness in the area where the hair was removed (don't get this done right before a date) and red bumps or breakouts in the area where the hair was removed. If you have oily skin or are prone to breakouts in the temple area, don't let the esthetician apply heavy creams to this area after waxing. The pores are open after hot wax has been applied, and the last thing you need to have is oily, greasy cream on your skin.

Another note of caution: If you are using any alpha hydroxy acid (AHA)-containing products, acne medications with Retin-A, or any other type of skin preparation that sloughs off the top layer of skin, refrain from their use for three to four days prior to waxing. The results of an eyebrow wax can be really ugly if you don't stop applying the cream ahead of time. Since the top layer of skin is being constantly, slightly abraded by the topical skin cream, getting a wax will literally rip off the loose layers of skin along with the hairs. The result can be a nasty scab that looks like a rug burn right along the eyebrow.

If you have never done your brows yourself, go to a salon frequented by a woman whose brows you know and love. Don't wander into a place because they have a sign outside advertising a special. You may be happy with the results, but in general it's a gamble. Try to go where you know they do good brows.

After you have achieved the shape you want with waxing or tweezing, you may have to finish off the brows with makeup. Women with ample eyebrow hair may not need any extras, but if you have short, sparse, or light-colored brows, eyebrow pencils or powder can be your best friend.

Polvo vs. Pencil

SINCE BROW PENCIL WEARS LONGER ON THE SKIN, USE ONE to fill in small areas of the brow where hair is sparse or on brows that don't have a lot of hair to begin with.

Powder adheres better to hair, so it is a better option for women who have substantial eyebrows and only want to fill in or extend the line of the brow. Powder is also the better choice when trying to change the color of the brow, which generally means going from a lighter-colored brow to a darker shade. Trying to go lighter doesn't work as well.

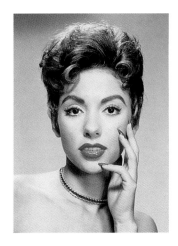

Un Tip **Rapidito**

Want to give yourself an eyebrow like Rita Moreno's in her West Side Story *days? New York City–based makeup artist José Parrón says you can create an arch that defies the laws of nature by using a pencil that matches your shade of brow color and gently, lightly extending the inner bottom corner of your eyebrow down slightly. When you do this on yourself, try it with one brow first. After you have extended the inner brow line of one eye, step back three to four feet from the mirror, and look at your reflection. By lowering the bottom of the inner corner, the midbrow appears to lift higher, creating the illusion of a more pronounced arch. Many women use a pencil on the high point of the arch to try and create lift. This rarely works. Go for the lower, inner brow, instead. You'll be amazed at the results.*

Pencil and powder are both great tools for defining brows. Add a coat of brow gel to keep the brow and the makeup in place throughout the day.

Técnica Tips

Learning how to make up your eyes the right way is like learning how to ride a bike: Once you master the basic technique for making your eyes look their best, you only have to adapt that technique to get a myriad of different looks. Lipstick colors change with the trends—what's in, what's out. But the basics of a good makeup application will always remain the same. Once you master a technique, you can adapt it to anything, changing colors from season to season, adding hue or intensity, or going from day to evening.

Learning what looks good on your pair of eyes, however, can be difficult and may be the reason so many women are reluctant to learn how to make them up fully. It's hard to be objective with yourself. When you see a makeup look that works on someone else, you can't just copy the look exactly. It needs to be adjusted to look right on you—on your eye color, on your eye shape. In fact, you can wear almost any look; you just have to personalize it. The differences depend on color choices, color intensity, and technique.

Lujoso vs. bueno, bonito, y barato

IN GENERAL, A GOOD BRUSH CAN RUN YOU IN the ballpark of $20–$30. An excellent one will cost in the mid-$20s. Before you buy, remember the rule of makeup money: If you use it often, it's worth it; if you don't, it's a waste. However, if you have never used a brush before, don't spend an exorbitant amount the first time around. Learn how to use the implement first and make it part of your routine. Then invest in a better one. As far as bristle content, only use natural-bristle brushes and try for sable, pony, or squirrel. These items can be purchased at department or cosmetics stores. And if you really want to indulge and you have the time and money to try the over-the-top eye looks we talk about later in this chapter, invest in each of the following tools.

Splurge
- All-over shadow brush
- Contour brush
- Powder eyeliner brush
- Liquid eyeliner brush

Save

Photocopy this list and take it with you to the drugstore. You can easily find excellent versions of these products there or at a beauty supply store.
- Eyelash curler
- Eyelash/brow brush
- Sponge-tip applicators
- Foundation sponges

Tools for making up your eyes

If you are really serious about eye makeup, the first step is to get the right tools. Investing in implements can also save money, since by using a great brush you can skimp on the quality of makeup and still look great. Brushes don't need to be outrageously expensive, but they do need to suit your needs. Consider the right brush to be an investment, not an expense. Once you develop a routine, you'll know which brushes will be worth investing in for you. Besides, as we'll show you later on, there are places where it's OK to save and others where it is worth it to splurge.

Cosas Necesarias

Here's what you need:

1. La mano. As in, your hands. The best makeup artists in the world carry a myriad of brushes, pencils, and powders to create beautiful faces, but the most important tools they have are their hands. Your hands, and more specifically, your fingers, are the tools you will use to blend and apply makeup. They are, therefore, the tools that enable you to express and bring out the beauty in your face. Think of using your hands on your face in the same way you use them when you massage your own feet or tired legs: It's an act of *cariño*. Your hands are your greatest beauty tools. Use them often.

2. All-over shadow brush. The size is larger than other eye brushes—about the size of your thumbnail—and the shape is usually round. In general, these brushes are used for applying light color all over the eyelid.

3. Eyelash curler. Some women look at it as a torture device, but women who know how to use one correctly don't leave home without it. It helps to lift the lash bed, opening up the eye. It allows you to get maximum definition without overusing mascara. And for women with straight-as-a-llama's lashes, curling provides an extra benefit: freedom from raccoon eyes, which can occur when you blink and mascara'd, uncurled lashes hit the undereye area, mixing with concealer. New curling-formula mascaras do give lashes a lift, but it can't compare to the beautiful, extended eye-opening effect created by one good squeeze with a curler.

4. Eyelash/brow brush. The two-sided comb/brushes you see at the drugstore can work, but you don't have to get that complicated; a toothbrush or spiral brush (the kind that looks like a mascara brush) and a fine-tooth comb can work just as well. Use them to groom the brows, to blend brow makeup, and to prevent clumping of eyelashes after mascara application.

5. Foundation sponge. Use this to clean up the undereye area by flicking away any remaining makeup debris that remains after the eye makeup application is complete.

6. Sponge-tip applicators. Use these when you want to apply light colors and build up opacity, since they give colors a heavier application. Avoid using them with dark colors.

7. Contour brush. No bigger than your pinky nail, this brush defines the eye by placing color in its smaller crevices. You can also use it to apply highlighter, although you will have to remove all excess powder when switching from a darker to lighter shade.

8. Powder eyeliner brush. Flat and small with stiff bristles, this brush lines the eyes by providing precise application of powder.

9. Liquid eyeliner brush. This has a tiny, pointed end, perfect for the exact definition and fine line that liquid eyeliner application requires. Most liquid eyeliners come with their own brush, but you will find that a longer-handled brush like this gives you more control.

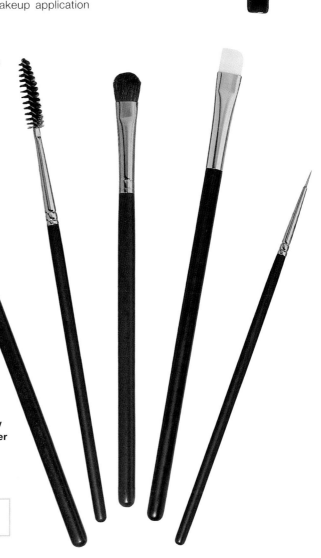

From left to right: All-over shadow brush, eyelash/brow brush, contour brush, powder eyeliner brush, and liquid eyeliner brush.

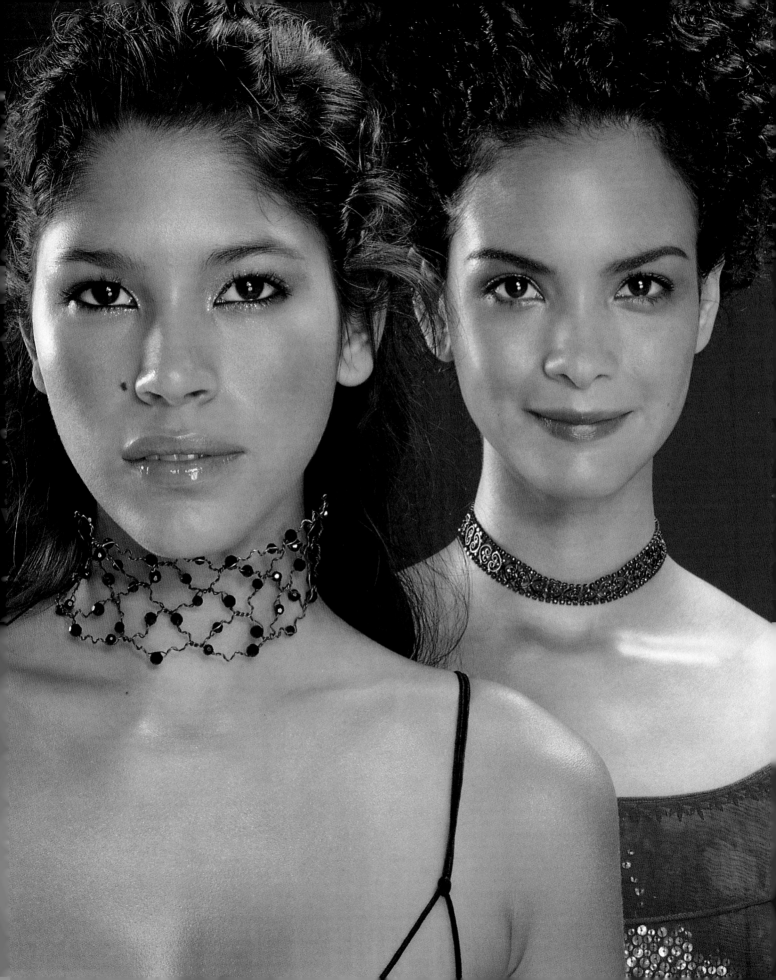

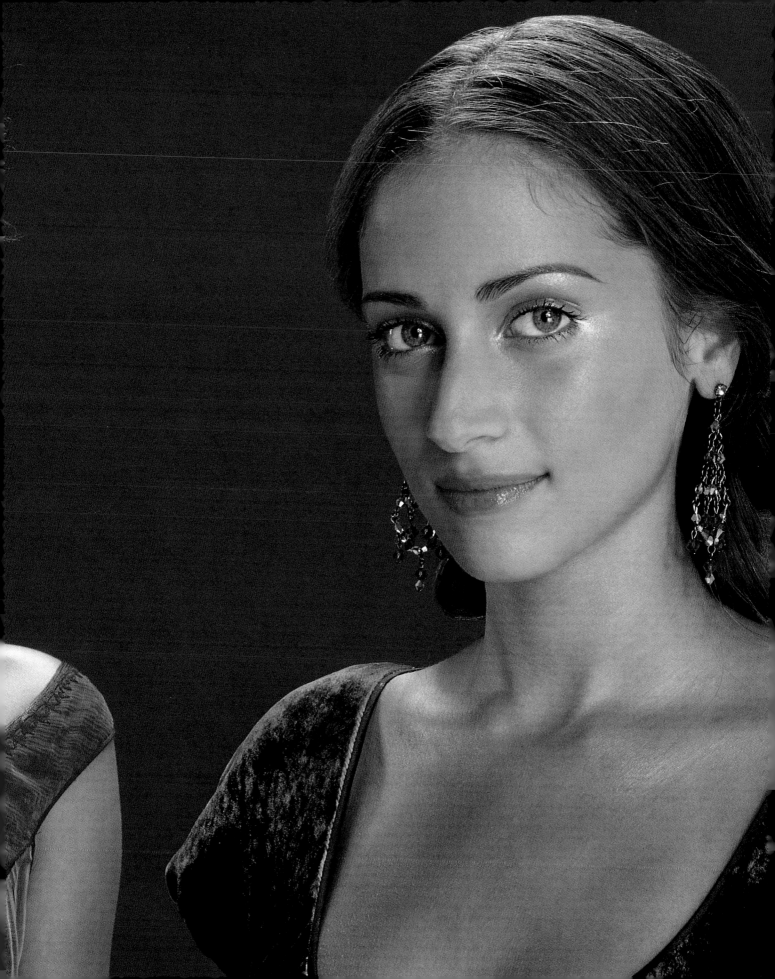

Different **Eye Looks**

The *Ahorita* Eye

The less-than-five-minute eye makeup look, for when you want to look pulled together but have better things to do than spend your time in front of a mirror.

• **Eye cream.** It may surprise you to find this here, but it's the first step in any eye makeup application. The eye area produces little to no oil, so it's up to us to keep it lubricated. This area also comprises the thinnest skin on the body. Invest in a good eye cream and, starting from the outer corner and working toward the nose, apply it with your ring finger, the finger that will place least pressure on this delicate skin.

• **Concealer.** This is one of the most important and misused beauty products. The first place you need to apply it is the inner corner of the eye, right next to the bridge, which is the darkest area around the eye. Use your fingers to dab on the concealer. You will be surprised at how little you need to brighten up the eye area. The less product you use the less likely it will be to clump and accumulate in the fine lines of the undereye area as well. Selecting the right concealer is tricky. Check out the sidebar below.

Concealer also evens out the tones and texture of the eyelid, creating a uniform canvas for eye-shadow application. Another of its functions is to maintain

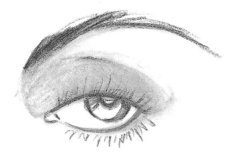

The *ahorita* eye uses a wash of lid color to give a quick, polished yet minimal makeup look. Experiment with different eye shadow colors and textures to vary the *ahorita* eye.

Concealer *consejos*

SELECTING THE RIGHT CONCEALER FOR THE undereye area requires more attention than most women think. Use a formula that "brightens" the eye area. A brightening concealer should reflect light, as opposed to giving opaque coverage over the skin. The difference is noticeable as the day wears on. A covering concealer masks the skin and looks fine upon first application, but by the end of the day it has disintegrated, broken up, and collected into the fine lines around the eye. A brightening concealer is translucent enough to show your natural skin as it blends fluidly in the eye area.

But for women with extremely dark circles— especially those with dark skin— the situation calls for something different. Using a concealer that is too light creates a grayish, ashy cast over the undereye area. The result is a tired, unhealthy look that actually draws attention to the problem instead of minimizing it. The solution: When choosing a concealer, select one that minimizes the darkness of the undereye area by blending it well with the face. This technique requires special attention to how you make up the rest of your skin. Choose a darker blush, for example, to maintain a smooth color transition in the area where you are essentially blending two skin tones; and select lighter colors for eye shadow, so as not to add to the darkness around the eye.

eye makeup and prevent creasing or sliding. For people with particularly oily skin, concealer helps eye makeup adhere and "hold on" to the lid. Again, use your finger in a light tapping motion to apply concealer on the lid, blending gently as you go along.

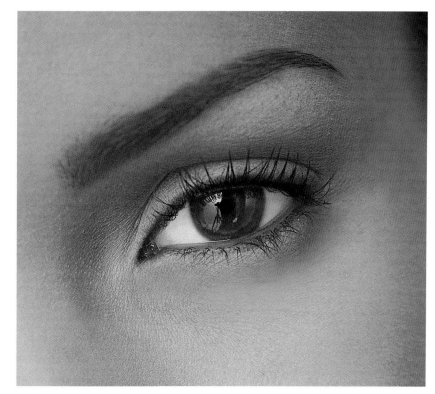

• **A basic all-over lid color.** A lid color should generally be a neutral, simple color you can apply over the entire eyelid to make your eyes look bright and awake. If you are daring, experiment with a color that has shimmer in the formula to reflect light and brighten the eye area. Another tip for *muchachas bravas*: Try a very subtle color wash, meaning that you select an eye shadow with color in it, but apply it sparingly to the eyelid. Try violet, light blue, white, or even green. The effect is fresh, youthful, and slightly funky. Apply this—in a neutral or bright color—with your all-over shadow brush.

• **Mascara.** Apply this after curling lashes with an eyelash curler. When investing in mascara, make sure it's the right formula for you. If you have sensitive eyes, purchase a formula that won't flake off or cause irritation. For daily wear, the best type of mascara is water resistant, especially in summer or if you live in a hot, humid climate, like parts of Texas and Florida. Waterproof mascara is very drying on the lashes and tends to start flaking by the time evening rolls around. Water-resistant mascara will stand up to the heat and to the natural oils produced by the skin in humid climates. If you have short, dense lashes, get a lengthening mascara. A thickening mascara is better for women whose lashes tend to be long but thin. For short, sparse lashes, a thickening mascara is also probably best, since it will help to build up the appearance of the lashes along the lash line, creating a nice fringe. Generally, select a black or dark brown color. We'll talk more about using different colors later.

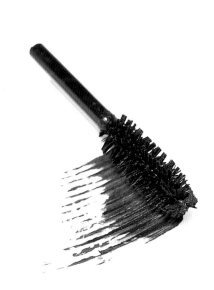

Did you know? Latinas are three times more likely than non-Hispanic women to apply mascara twice a day.

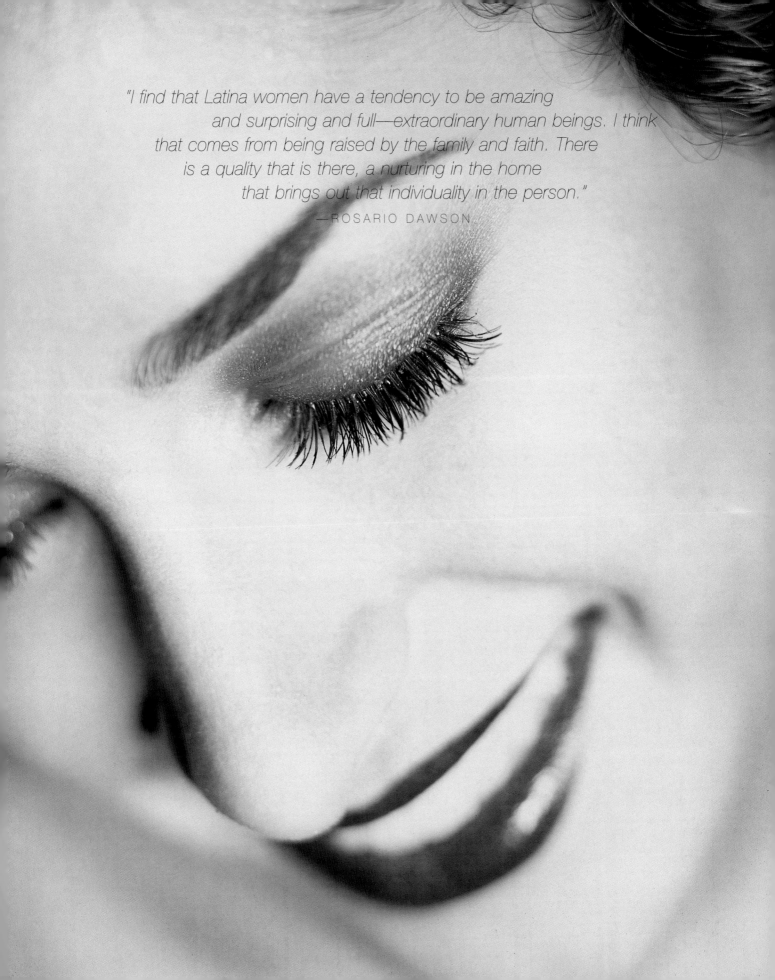

"I find that Latina women have a tendency to be amazing and surprising and full—extraordinary human beings. I think that comes from being raised by the family and faith. There is a quality that is there, a nurturing in the home that brings out that individuality in the person."

—ROSARIO DAWSON

The *Diez Minutitos* Eye

For evening and for special occasions when you have the luxury of time and want to indulge yourself, the *diez minutitos* eye employs techniques of shading and highlighting. For all you aspiring artists out there, here's an opportunity to create shape using light and dark, with your face as the canvas. After you have applied the basic, all-over eyelid color, take these next steps to make your eyes really *hacer el empeño*.

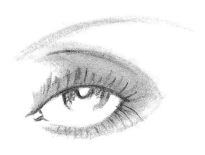

• **Contour shadow.** Choose a darker-colored eye shadow to apply to the crease of the eye, and be certain to draw your contour brush across the eye-shadow pan so that its bristles pick up an adequate amount of powder. Excess powder can be removed by tapping the brush over the eye-shadow pan. Work from the outer toward the inner corner of the eye. If you are doing this for the first time, try this technique: Holding a mirror in one hand, position the mirror so that your face is angled down slightly but your eyes are looking up at the mirror. Keep your eyes open, take the contour brush with your dominant hand, and apply the contour shadow along the brow bone where your open eye meets the crease.

At first, you may find it difficult to apply shadow exactly along the crease. Don't worry, because after creating this line along the crease you can use your all-over eye-shadow brush to blend well. This technique is good for women whose eyes are well spaced apart. If your eyes are very close together, apply contour shadow on the outer crease only. Drawing the crease toward the inner eye will only create a dark space between the eyes, making them look even closer together.

• **Highlighter shadow.** A highlighter shadow is a color that is lighter than either the all-over lid color or the contour shadow. Use your contour brush to apply the highlighter along the brow bone up to the eyebrow. (Make sure, of course, that any remnants of the contour shadow have been tapped off or wiped off the bristles with a tissue.) The highlighter brightens the overall look of the eye. If your eyes are close together, it is also a good idea to apply highlighter at the inner eye area along the top lash line. This draws light toward the inner eye area, creating the illusion of more space between the two eyes. For many women, the *diez minutitos* eye can stop right here, needing only a quick curl of the eyelashes and a coat of mascara.

• **Eyeliner.** Even more than eye shadow, eyeliner is an easy way to really change the look of the eye. There are a lot of different kinds of eyeliner, and when it comes to liquid eyeliner many women are reluctant to experiment. For this particular look, we'll just talk about the easiest form to work with—eye shadow used as eyeliner.

Lid color

Highlighter

Contour shadow/
eyeliner shadow

The *diez minutitos* eye can be created with neutrals to contour and give shape and depth, or it can be used with dramatic eye makeup (below) for more impact. Paired with individual false lashes (left) the *diez minutitos* eye transforms into the *¡dale niña!* eye and commands attention.

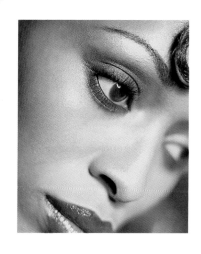

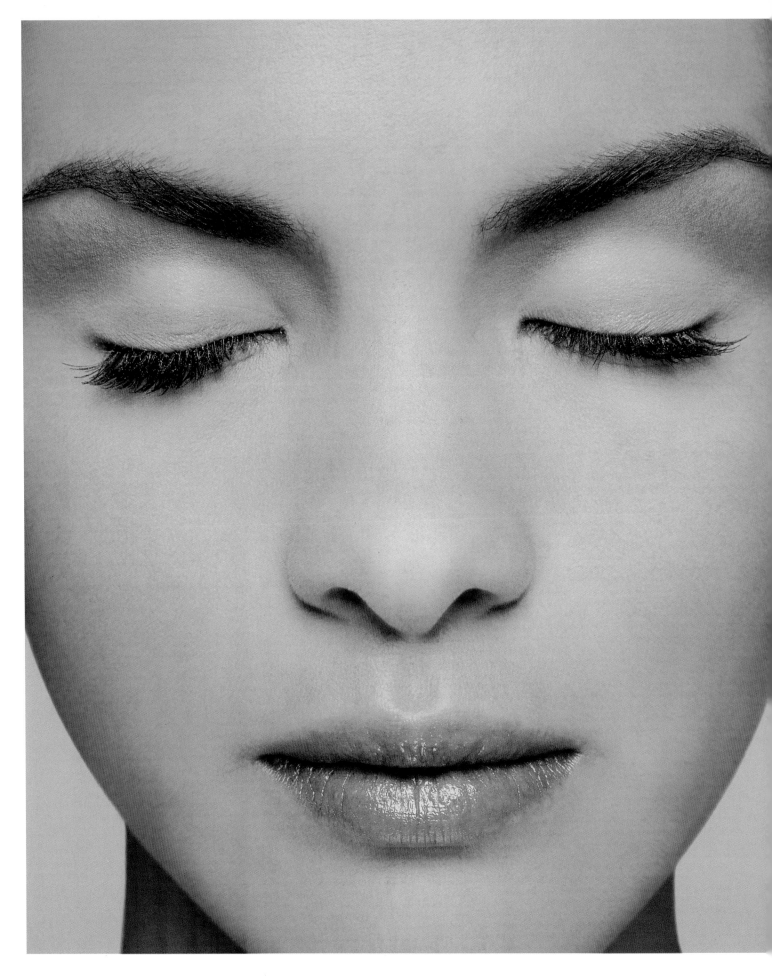

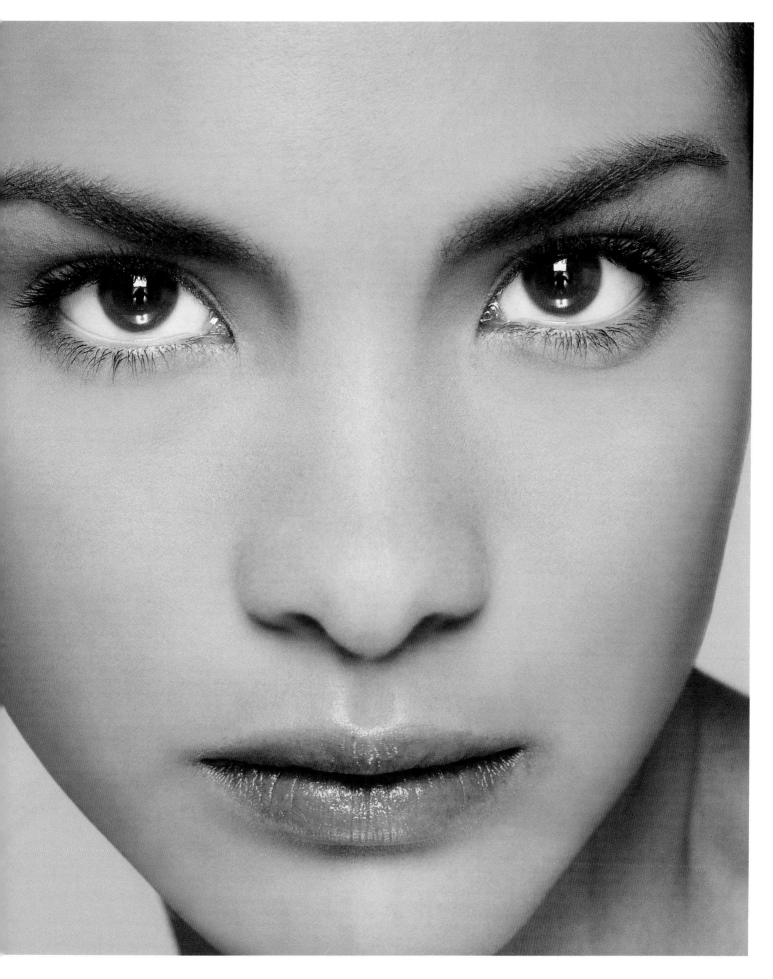

Eyeliner defines the eye, but too much can make the eye appear smaller. The unlined eye (near right) looks rounder and larger, while the heavily lined eye (far right) looks dramatic and smoky—still beautiful but slightly smaller.

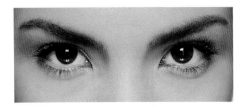

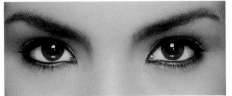

Un Tip *Rapidito*

If you absolutely cannot give up your eyeliner pencil, at least try to get the right kind. A good consistency is not too hard and not too soft. The test: Drag the pencil tip along the back of your hand. If the lead breaks, or tugs at the skin, it is too hard, and maybe too old. Throw it out. If the pencil lead mushes into the skin or leaves thick globs instead of a smooth line, it is too oily and will probably run after only a few hours of wear. Throw this one out too. The line should draw on the skin fluidly, without requiring excessive pressure or resulting in excess liner smeared on the skin.

We'll also be honest with you and tell you what you won't read in other beauty books: A harsh line, whether drawn with liquid or pencil, actually makes the eye look smaller. Lining the inner rim of the lower lash line, in particular, makes the eyes noticeably smaller. This may rock your eyeliner-dependent world, and giving up your pencil may feel like going through withdrawal. (That thick black stripe drawn along the top lash line is also a common mistake—we've been there.) But just suspend disbelief and listen: Using eye shadow imparts a softer line, opening up the eyes instead of shutting them down.

Use a powder eyeliner brush and dark eye shadow to line the eye. Start by dipping the brush in the eye-shadow pan, again, drawing it across to pick up enough powder on its bristles and then tapping it over the eye-shadow pan to remove excess powder. Apply the shadow by placing and slightly pressing the edges of the brush bristles as close to the top lash line as possible. After applying slight pressure, lift the brush and move it over to the next section. It's almost like creating a dotted line across the lash line, except the dots are so close together, they are connected. You don't brush the line on, the way you would the rest of the shadows—you dot it on, building up enough pigment to create a continuous line. Start by applying a thick application to the outside, upper lash line, as close to the lashes as possible, making it thinner as you work toward the inner eye area. Draw your line over the outer two-thirds of the eye only. If you are not yet expert at applying eyeliner and making one eye even with the other, smudge the line using a cotton swab or a sponge-tip

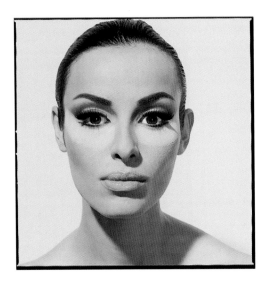

Un Tip *Rapidito*

Here is a trick makeup artists use at photo shoots when they are applying heavy or dramatic eye makeup on models, and one you should consider when you are about to apply complicated, heavy makeup on yourself. It's certainly not necessary for everyday use. While the technique is not new— it's from back in the '60s, when women went all out and spared no eye makeup detail—it really works. Before starting to apply eye makeup, dab a generous amount of loose powder on the undereye area. This powder will be used to "catch" any excess dark eye shadow that may fall from the bristles of the eye-shadow brush as you apply color. When you are done applying color to the eyes, use a large fluffy powder brush to brush away the excess loose powder, taking away with it any eye shadow that has fallen underneath the eye area.

applicator. Smudging creates a softer, sexy line and is a great technique for hiding mistakes. Again, do this only on the outer two-thirds of the top lash line. After applying the eyeliner, curl your lashes, apply the mascara, and you are ready to go.

The *¡Dale Niña!* Eye

This is where we have fun—the outlandish fake-eyelash, liquid-eyeliner eye, which can be used to impress or to shock. I recommend trying this out at least once a year. Why let movie stars have all the fun?

Sit down at a table where you can rest your elbows comfortably. Take a large-size handheld mirror in the hand you don't write with and the liquid eyelining brush in the other. Keep your head held high, but lower the hand mirror until your eyes must look down to see into it. Anchor your other elbow (the one with the hand holding the eyeliner brush) on the tabletop so your hand will be steady. Bring the hand with the eyeliner brush to your face. Rest the pinky finger on the cheek directly under the eye to be lined; then, gripping the lining brush with your pointer finger and thumb, lightly draw the line starting at the outer edge of the upper lash line. Draw it as close to the lash line and as thinly as possible. Don't try to draw a thick line at once, because the idea is to thicken the line gradually so you won't be stuck with one fat, ungraceful line. The goal with liquid eyeliner is to create a line that is thicker at the outer edges, becoming thinner as it goes toward the inner eye, until it becomes extremely thin at the inner corner. Most women don't even try to line the entire upper lash line, since it's just too hard to get it right. Instead, they line the outer two-thirds, which generally looks better anyway. As you become more adept at this application, you probably won't need to rest your elbows on a table.

Not only for the sure-of-hand, liquid eyeliner can be applied expertly by all—*con tiempo* and plenty of practice.

Many hermanas *complain about liquid eyeliner clumping their eyelashes when they try applying it. This can be especially irritating if you have naturally curly or very long lashes to begin with. Looking down helps minimize any potential tangling by keeping the lashes down and out of the way. If you get some of the liquid tangled up in the lashes anyway, don't fret, simply use the fine-tooth eyelash comb to separate them after the liquid has dried. Curl the lashes, and apply less mascara than you normally would—liquid eyeliner does get caught up in the base of the lash line, so adding mascara from the roots to the tips as you normally do would simply leave a thick, globby mess.*

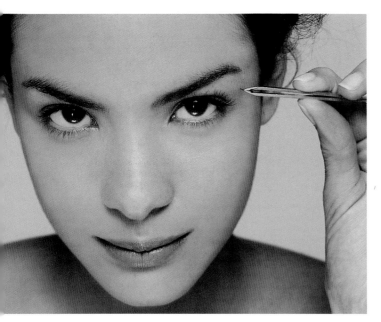

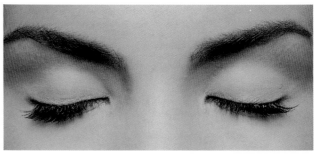

Bunches of individual lashes not only create more length but can help to fill a sparse lash line. Trim the false lashes to match you own length before applying. Then, anchor each lash bunch along the lash line on bare spots or areas where lashes are thin.

Since liquid eyeliner makes such a strong impact visually, most women can simply curl the eyelashes, add a coat of mascara, and call it a day. But why not go for the all-out glamour? Add about three or four bunches of individual false lashes to the outer corners of the eyelash line, after you have applied the liquid eyeliner. Using a pair of tweezers, pick up one bunch of individual lashes near, but not exactly at, the base. Dip the base in the eyelash adhesive, and place the base at the outer edge of the top lash line. Hold the lashes there, applying slight pressure for a count of ten to fifteen seconds. Then release the tweezers. The lashes should have adhered to the eyelid. Place the next bunch beside the first, working toward the inner eye. Use only three to four bunches, since you are looking for a flirty, cat-eye effect. You may want to finish by adding more liquid eyeliner over the upper edge where the lashes have been glued. Be very careful, though, as longer lashes can make eyeliner application a bit trickier.

Beautiful Brown Eyes

Make your brown eyes woo

The biggest tragedy surrounding Latina beauty is how many of us with brown eyes accept the outdated (and dare we say jealousy-inspired) adage that brown eyes are boring. This cliché has been extended to a near edict that they be made up only with brown eye shadow, or maybe a bronze color once in a while. In fact, if you listen to most beauty magazines' eye-shadow color stories, light eyes come in a variety of shades—gray, green, blue, hazel, dark green, etc.— while brown eyes are simply, well, brown. These magazines need to visit our *barrios* more often. If they did, they would know there are many types of brown eyes and no shortage of Latinas willing to experiment with eye-shadow colors. If you want to experiment with your eye makeup to bring out the gold flecks, to change your brown to a mesmerizing, almost gold-green color, or to heighten the impact of your already beautiful deep brown, almost black eyes, the key is knowing which colors to try.

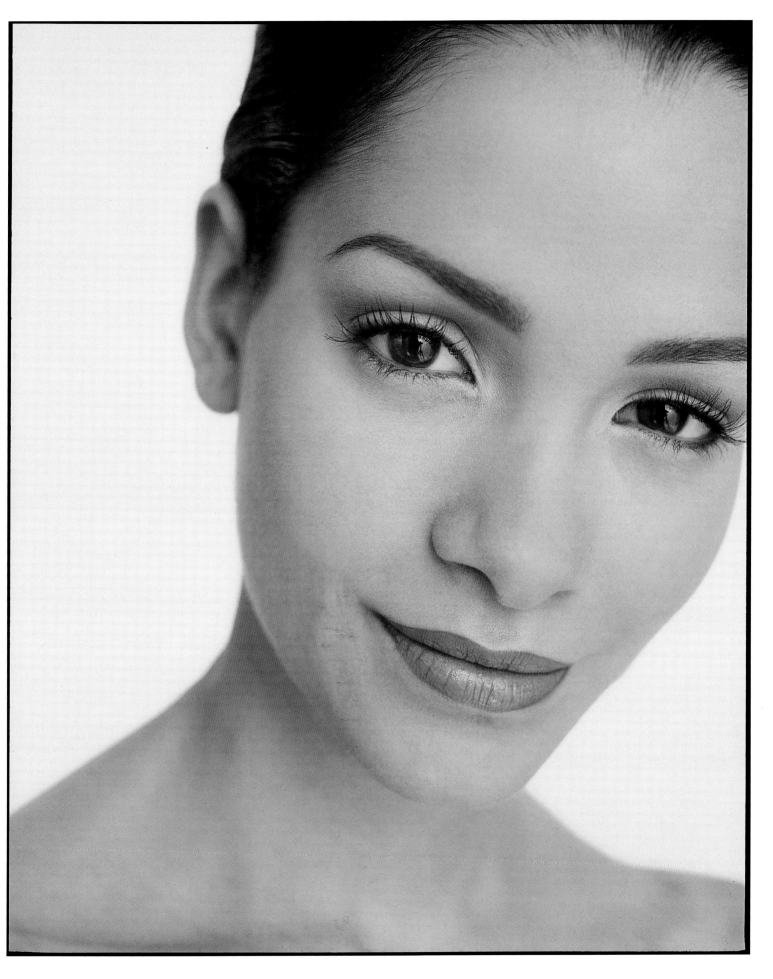

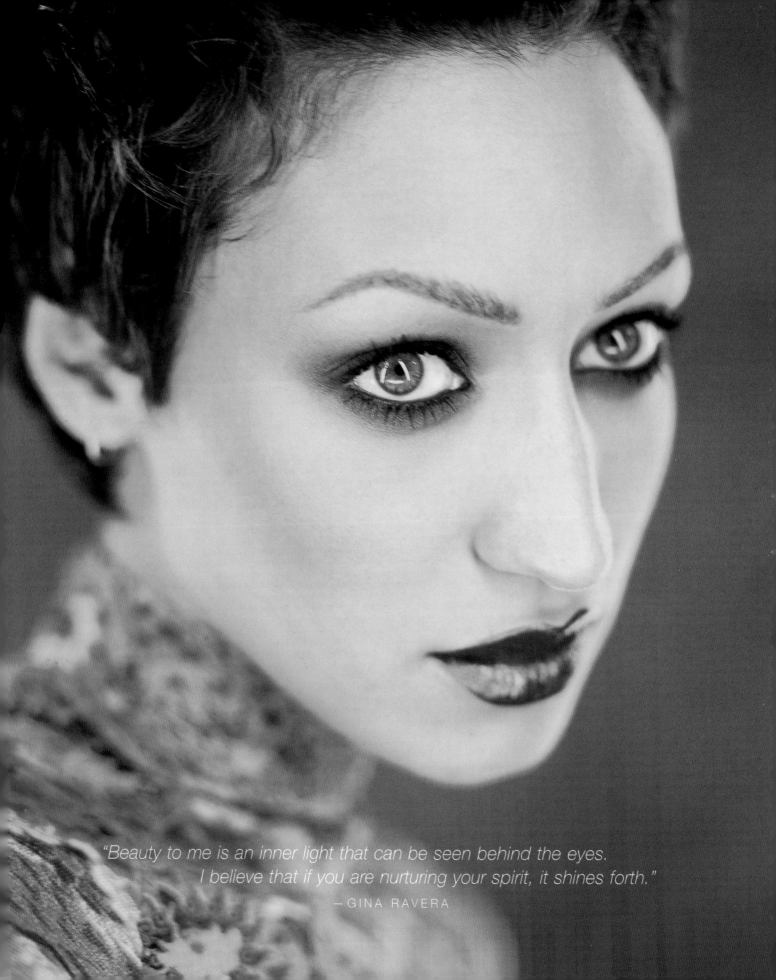

"Beauty to me is an inner light that can be seen behind the eyes.
I believe that if you are nurturing your spirit, it shines forth."
— GINA RAVERA

Using the color wheel

You remember the color wheel. It was what you learned about in kindergarten when your teacher was trying to get you to mix paints. The colors weren't placed on the wheel just any old way. They were placed in relation to each other. Yellow, red, and blue are the primary colors. Yellow and red mixed together make orange, so orange appears between red and yellow on the wheel. Red and blue mixed together make purple, so purple lies between them, and blue and yellow mixed together make green, so green falls between them. Did you make your own color wheel in kindergarten? Well, here is something your kindergarten teacher may not have told you: The color wheel also works so that each color on the wheel brings out or accentuates the color directly opposite.

CHART

A todo color

Color you want to emphasize	Color opposite on the wheel	Eye makeup color to use
Green	Red	**Pink, bronze, champagne**
Yellow	Purple	**Violet, maroons, burgundy**
Gold	Blue and purple	**Navy blue, blue-gray, bright blue**
Gray	Yellow and orange	**Gold, amber, russet**

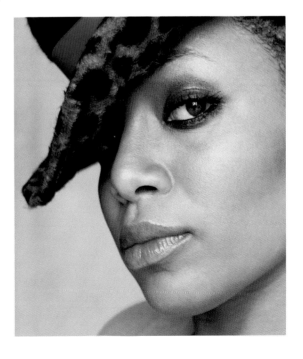

A smoky effect in vibrant purple brings out the depth of brown eyes.

Why should you care about this, and what does it have to do with eye makeup? If you want to bring out certain flecks in your eyes, apply the color wheel theory to your selection of eye shadows. For example, say you want to bring out green flecks in your brown eyes. The color opposite green on the wheel is red. Does this mean you run out and purchase red eye shadow? No, you would look sick. What it means is you can experiment with eye shadows that have red tones in them: Pinks, roses, even purples—all of these will bring out the green flecks or green hue in your eyes. See the chart above for a complete rundown.

You can use these colors both in terms of the eyeliners you choose and for the mascaras you select. These tools give you a cast of colors that bring out the effect you want without the obviousness an eye shadow can have.

This principle applies if you also want to emphasize your brown eyes by intensifying the brown or by giving them an ebony cast. In this case, since you are emphasizing the color they already are, you would go with colors that deepen, not contrast. So apply rich chocolate browns, deep charcoal grays, and black. Still doubtful? Check out these different types of brown-eyed women and how we made their *ojos* pop.

Retro-Latina Eye Looks

Rita Hayworth • '40s Screen Siren

Rita Hayworth (whose real name was Margarita Cansino) perfected the *¡dale niña!* eye with a strip of extra-long, obviously fake lashes. The big difference: She also had her own full, thick brows tweezed to an extremely thin line and extended the eyebrow line with eyebrow pencil. (No, they didn't grow that long naturally.) Paired with *rojo sangre* lips and flawless skin—a gift of great lighting and heavy pancake makeup along with really good genes—Rita was ready. Her look, while highly dramatic thanks to the fake lashes, is more classical.

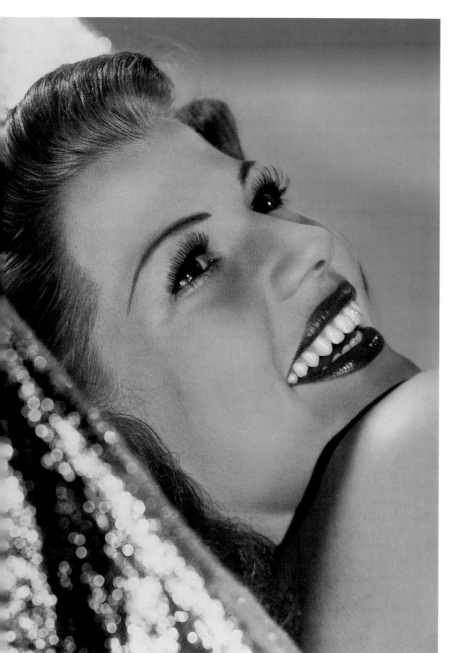

Raquel Welch • '70s Pinup Eyes

Raquel Welch, whose father was Bolivian, was the international sex symbol of her day. In the late '60s to early '70s, she personified femininity, sex appeal, and adventurousness. Her eyes were done up in a cross between the *diez minutitos* eye and the *¡dale niña!* Contouring was used in the crease to give her eyes a smoky depth, and liquid eyeliner was used for dramatic impact. The eyeliner was extended beyond the eye, but the upper and lower lines never meet. This prevents the eye from looking too enclosed by the heavy eye makeup. Another Raquel beauty secret: White eyeliner was applied on the bottom inner rim of the eye. This creates a wide-open, bigger-looking eye. But do a reality check before trying this on yourself. While white eyeliner looks good at first, liner applied to the inner rim causes the eye to water slightly—its natural reaction to contact with a foreign substance—and after a few hours can wind up as white gunk in the inner corner of the eye. Also, Latinas with dark eyelashes must apply the pencil very carefully. If you get some particles of the liner caught or rubbed into the base of the lower eyelashes, it looks like you have white stuff stuck to your lashes. Unsightly, to say the least.

Raquel finishes this highly made-up look with light lipstick paired with a tiny line of dark lipliner. Over all, this represents a very trendy look for the time.

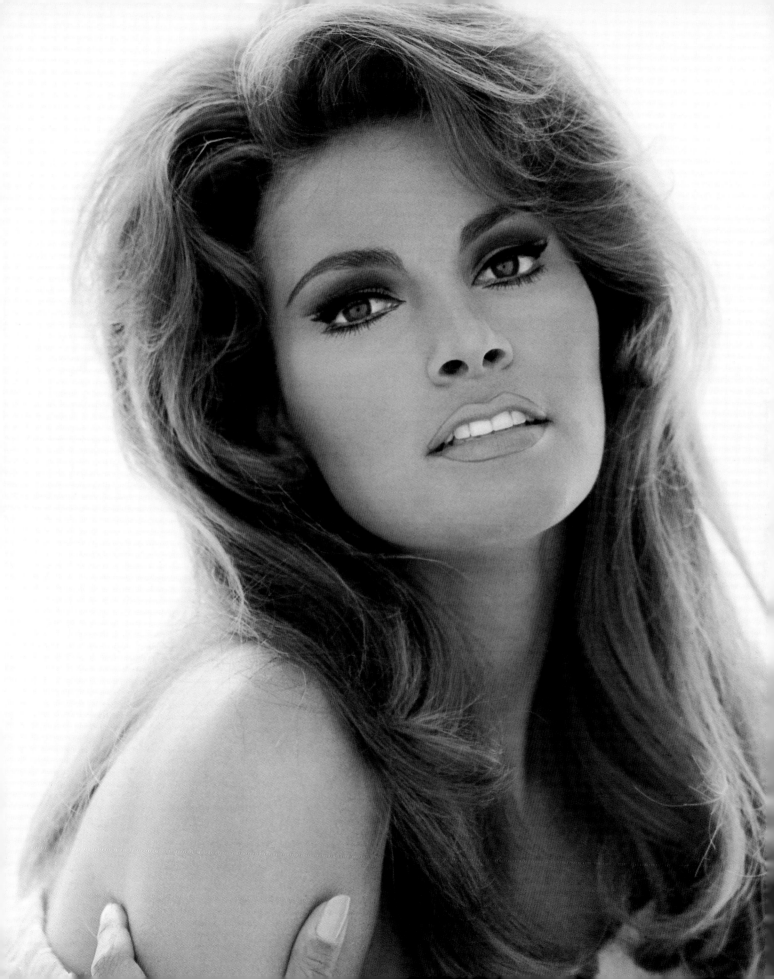

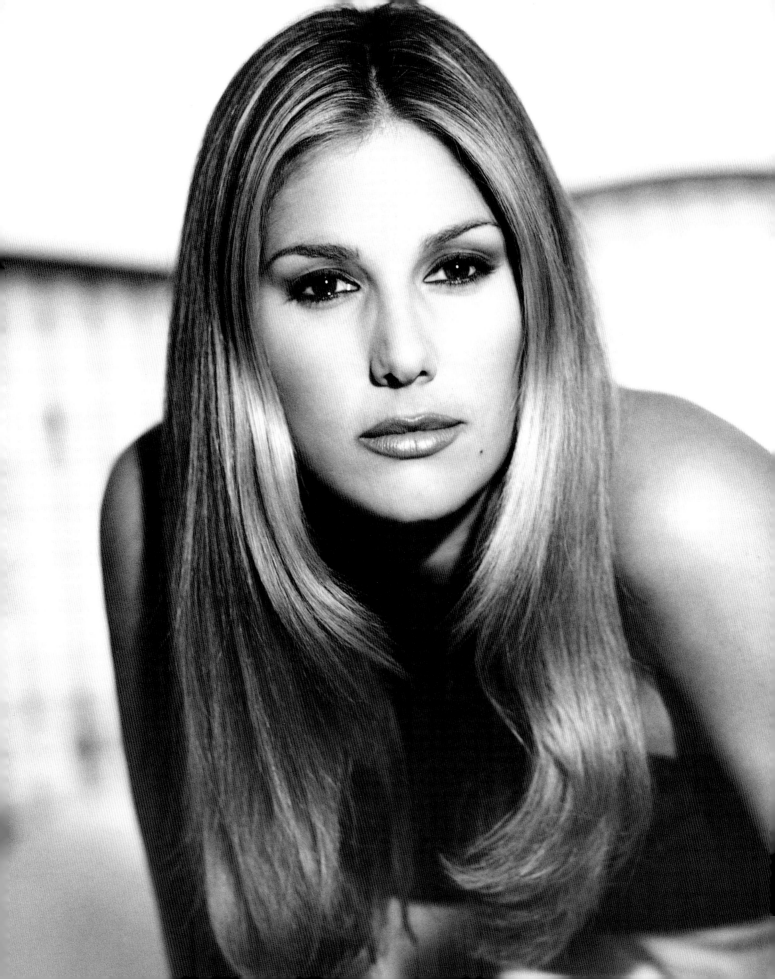

Silky, Curly, Sexy, Straight:
Your Crowning Glory

LATINA HAIR KNOWS NO SINGLE DEFINITION EXCEPT "BEAUtiful." Along with our skin tones, the texture of our hair can really run the gamut—from a headful of gorgeous *rizos* to luxurious curtains of sleek, straight locks. The hair colors bestowed upon us by nature are equally diverse, as are the colors we are *brava* enough to give ourselves: We are definitely not afraid to experiment. After all, isn't it true that Latinas never go gray, we just "evolve" into redheads?

Fortunate enough to have arrived at an era that happily embraces all our hair textures, we have liberated ourselves from dated notions of *pelo bueno, pelo malo,* and *pelo indio.* Each hair type has its own unique beauty, and we respond accordingly by caring for it appropriately.

Keeping It **Natural**

HAIR KEPT IN ITS NATURAL TEXTURE AND COLOR IS BY FAR THE EASI-est type to keep beautiful and healthy. Regular washing, conditioning, and trims are all that is needed.

Cleaning

Good shampoos must perform two important functions that are sometimes at odds: They must thoroughly clean the hair while not stripping away its protective oils.

Conditioning

Labor-intensive deep-conditioning treatments are not a necessary part of the regular routine for people who keep their hair natural. But if you style your hair with heat implements regularly, you may find you need a deep-conditioning treatment anywhere from once a week to once a month to maintain your hair's health.

Rizado

• Curly hair tends to be drier than straight hair. Be sure to condition the hair regularly after you shampoo. Sleeping on a satin pillowcase can also help by allowing your tresses to retain the natural oils secreted by your scalp. A satin pillowcase also reduces matting and frizz.

• Use styling products that are light and liquid. These will enhance and hold the curl without weighing the hair down.

• Even though it is less obvious than with straight hair, curly hair needs to be trimmed regularly, every six to ten weeks, just like straight hair. A dead giveaway of needing a trim: curls that frizz rather than "hold" at the ends of your hair.

Mami says: "Brush your hair a hundred times a day to help it grow fast and keep it soft and shiny."

Beauty myth **busted!**

Stylist says: It depends on your hair. Lilia Corvera, who owns Sherwood Hair Design, in Odessa, Texas, cautions that this old trick can actually damage some *cabellos*. "This practice is meant to moisturize hair by circulating your own natural oils. But if you have chemically treated—curly-permed, dyed/highlighted, or relaxed—hair, or very curly or textured hair, the ends are fragile and might break with excessive brushing."

Dry hair/oily scalp: The hair-care solution

WHAT IF YOU HAVE AN OILY SCALP, BUT DRY hair? What if your hair's dryness is compounded by its having been chemically treated, making frequent shampooing not such a good idea?

• Pick your shampoo for your scalp, not your hair type. Look for formulas that are meant for fine/limp hair, or specifically for oily hair. These shampoos have detergents that effectively remove excess oil.

• Before washing your hair, apply conditioner to the ends to protect them from the harsh detergents in the shampoo. Don't worry about not being able to clean the ends; the shampoo runs off your hair as you rinse, and the lather cleanses the ends.

• Apply shampoo to the scalp only, using your hands to make sure the product is spread evenly.

• Select a conditioner for your hair type. Get an extra-moisturizing conditioner, but apply it only where you need it: from midlength to the ends. Avoid getting conditioner on or near your scalp.

• Keep any greasy styling products, like hair-dressing creams or pomades, on the ends, away from the roots.

• To extend your wash for a day, apply witch hazel with a cotton ball to your scalp. Other options to absorb excess oil: Dry shampoo, essentially powder in a spray bottle, allows you to spray the roots with powder that absorbs oil; natural-bristle brushes distribute excess oil further down the hair shaft.

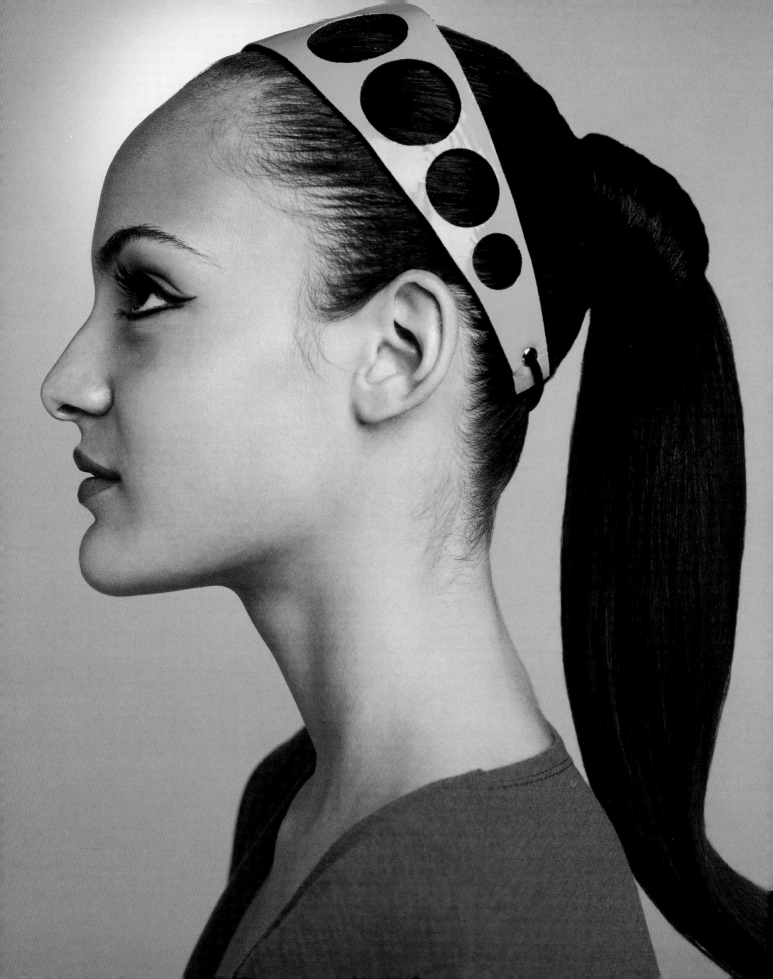

Largo

Long hair is old hair, and as such needs special care. Although there are a few products on the market specially designed for long hair, all you really need to do is the following:

- Spot-apply moisturizing products like leave-in conditioner or hairdressing cream to the ends.
- Pomades and silicon drops should also be applied to the ends.
- Don't expect to defy gravity. Long hair is also very heavy. Teasing up a headful of high, long hair is fine for *telenovela* actresses and beauty queens, or for a special occasion. But unless you cut in layers to create more body or are ready to tease, spray, and damage the hair every day, expect to have hair that pretty much lies flat at the crown.
- If you have long hair or are trying to grow it long and you also treat it chemically, you need to be extra gentle. On days you are at home, pull your hair back into a ponytail and apply conditioner to the ponytail, concentrating especially on the ends.
- Applying conditioner is also a great idea if you are going to be exercising or spending a day at the beach. The heat from your body or the sun plus the conditioner makes for an instant deep-conditioning treatment.

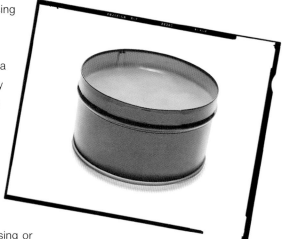

Old-school beauty products, like this hair pomade, aren't just for your *abuela*. Pomade helps to smooth ends.

Hair **Styling**

FOR A LOT OF US, "WASH-AND-GO" HAIR IS SIMPLY NOT A REALITY. Whether we keep it natural, wear it curly, or blow it straight, we prefer to style our hair. Some methods are better than others. While there are no miracles for quick-and-easy styling (except one: The shorter the hair, the shorter the styling time) there are more effective ways to get the look you are trying to achieve.

Blow-drying hair straight

If you frequently blow-dry your hair straight, here are a few tips to keep it looking healthy and fabulous.

✔ When you can, use heat-protective products. These truly useful products can help extend the time between trims. Some women find that using a heat-protective shampoo and conditioner leaves their hair slightly flat after styling. Try using one or the other instead of both at the same time. Experiment until you find what works best for you.

✔ The more you blow-dry, the more you are likely to need to incorporate a deep-conditioning treatment into your regular hair-care routine. Even with the advances of heat-protective and -activated hair-care and styling products, nothing can replace a good old-fashioned deep-conditioning treatment.

✔ Get regular trims. Frayed and split ends are especially noticeable on straight

Did you know? Latinas are 39 percent more likely than non-Hispanic women to use conditioner 4 or more times per week.

hair. You may notice that if you blow-dry your hair straight frequently, a month or so after a trim the ends begin to get a little frizzy, no matter what product you apply. This is your hair letting you know it needs a trim. Do it before the ends split, since afterward they may require a more drastic trim than you want.

✔ Heat-styling the hair straight exposes it to a lot of stress. Inevitably, wiry, short hairs will spring up around your part near the roots, where they break off due to excessive pulling and stretching. The best way to tame these coiled frizzies is to smooth on a light coating of styling gel, starting from the part.

✔ You may already use straightening or smoothing products with silicon, which are very effective in preventing frizz and keeping the hair cuticle smooth. But it is a better idea to use moisturizing styling products, such as hairdressing creams, directly after a trim and save the silicon-based products for when the hair has started to frizz slightly and you are closer to needing the next trim. This technique ensures that you are being as gentle to your hair as possible for as long as possible, before bringing out the silicon, which has little to no moisturizing properties.

Tools

• **Large, round, boar-bristle brush.** Select size by testing that the length of the hair wraps around the brush only once. If it wraps around twice, you need a bigger brush that won't get caught up in the hair. Obviously, if you have very long hair, it will wrap around any brush more than once. In this case, purchase the largest brush available.

Sectioning and separating makes hair infinitely easier to blow straight.

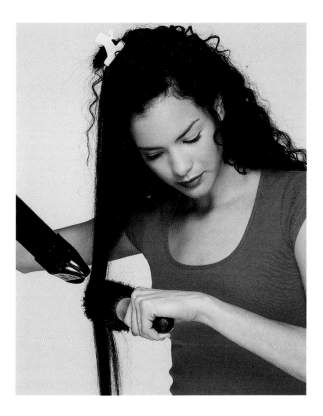

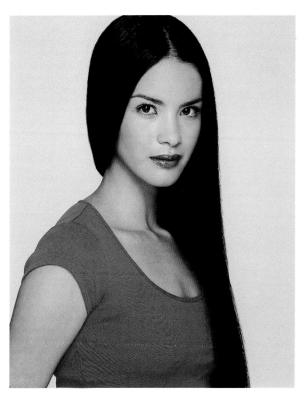

A great brush has just the right amount of grip and slide: The bristles grip the hair so it is pulled taut and straight, yet there is enough slide that you can draw the brush through the hair. The grip of the bristles should be chosen according to your hair type; *mujeres* with hair that is more wavy than curly will need a brush with a tighter grip. The grip of the bristles is generally affected by the stiffness of the bristles. Don't go overboard. If you have a headache—or a neck ache—from trying to keep your head up as you pull your hair straight, you need a softer brush.

- **Round aluminum brush (optional).** The advantage to aluminum brushes is that the inner core warms with the heat of the dryer, providing a styling and heat double whammy. They can be used in place of or in addition to a boar-bristle brush, especially on hard-to-straighten areas like the crown of the head or bangs.
- **Hair clips.** Dividing the hair and sectioning off areas you have dried from areas you have yet to dry is essential, especially if you are a blow-drying novice.
- **Long-tail teasing comb.** Use this to make clear parts as you section the hair.
- **Wide-tooth comb.** This is for combing and evenly distributing product throughout the hair.
- **Professional blow-dryer.** Available at beauty supply stores, professional dryers have a higher wattage (from 1,500 to 1,875, the highest available) than blow-dryers available at drugstores (around 1,200). Professional dryers also have more options in terms of heat and air-speed settings. Some also come equipped with a cold-shot button, which you can use to seal the cuticle down smoothly for extra shiny, straight hair. The most important feature of a professional dryer is a nozzle attachment that targets the air into a smaller area, an absolute must for blow-drying hair straight. This allows you to target air and heat directly to the brush as you straighten.
- **Hair-straightening balm.** Use a wide-tooth comb to distribute balm evenly over the entire head of hair.
- **Hairdressing cream.** These creams preserve moisture in extra-curly or damaged hair, which is put at risk for even greater damage by excessive heat. If your hair is dry but not extremely curly, a good option is to apply hairdressing cream only to the ends. Creams are heavier styling tools, so apply with a light hand.
- **Pomade or silicon drops (optional).** Hairdressing creams should eliminate the need for these, but pomades and silicon drops can impart extra smoothing

Clockwise, starting from top: A large, round brush and an oval paddle brush, an aluminum brush, wide-tooth comb, long-tail teasing comb, blow-dryer with straightening nozzle, and hair clips.

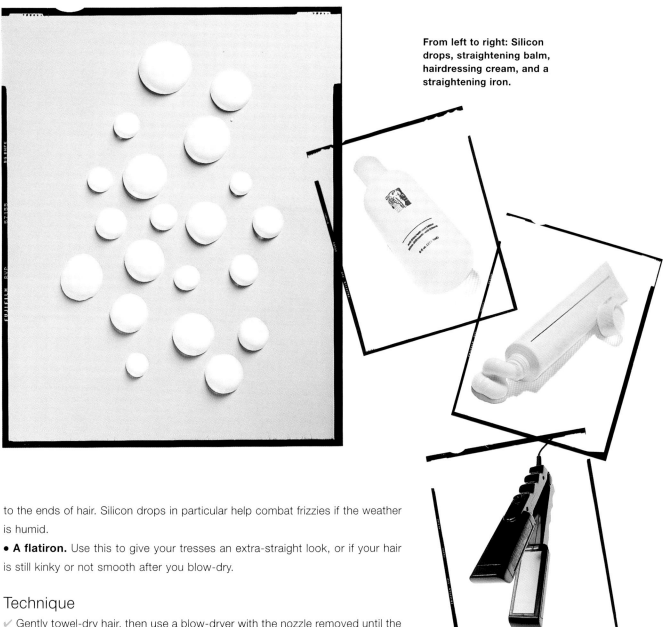

From left to right: Silicon drops, straightening balm, hairdressing cream, and a straightening iron.

to the ends of hair. Silicon drops in particular help combat frizzies if the weather is humid.

• **A flatiron.** Use this to give your tresses an extra-straight look, or if your hair is still kinky or not smooth after you blow-dry.

Technique

✔ Gently towel-dry hair, then use a blow-dryer with the nozzle removed until the hair is no longer soaking wet. Latinas with a looser curl or wave to their hair should dry until damp, minimizing the amount of direct heat hair gets subjected to in the styling process. For *hermanas* with a tighter curl, though, the hair is more pliable when it is wet, so you will have to resort to the direct heat sooner.

✔ Apply the straightening balm and the cream on dry ends, if needed. Heat-protective styling products are also an excellent choice.

✔ Divide hair into two-to-three-inch sections, using clips to secure the hair you are not working on. Begin with the sections in the back. Blow-drying your entire head can be hard on the arms, and the back of the head is the toughest part to get to. Do that area at the beginning and the rest is pretty easy. Be warned: Underlying layers that are not dried properly and remain damp will result in frizzy hair.

Remedios caseros

Scent saver:
Rub a few drops of vanilla extract in the palms of your hands, then smooth the palms over your hair to rid your pelo of smoky smells.

✔ Place the large round brush at the base of the hair section close to the scalp, and situate the dryer so that the brush is parallel to the nozzle. This will ensure that the heat hits the hair evenly. Run the brush down the length of the hair, following with the dryer. You may have to redo certain areas, like the ends. After you think a section is completely dry, check for dampness by pressing your palm against it. Your hair should be pretty much bone-dry before you move on to the next section.

✔ For areas where you want more lift or body, such as the crown, be sure to position the hair upward, away from the head, as you dry. Make sure the roots in particular are dried in this fashion. Applying a volumizing spray to the roots before drying also helps.

✔ After you are done drying the entire head of hair, use hairdressing cream, pomade, or silicon drops. Apply a small amount to your hands, rub between the palms, and apply to the ends only. Silicon will help seal and smooth the fragile ends. Don't go overboard with these products, since too much moisture and humidity are the enemies of blown-out hair.

What does it mean when I see steam rising from my hair dryer?

"It's the products you have used on your hair burning away," says celeb stylist to the stars Oribé, who is responsible for the locks of Jennifer Lopez, Salma Hayek, Penélope Cruz, and Gloria Estefan. The humidity of the damp hair meeting with the hot air of the dryer increases the likelihood of steam. Not to worry, though. As long as it's just the product, Oribé assures us, our tresses are safe. "If you smell your hair burning, then you're in trouble."

Doing *El Doobie*

The doobie was born back in the days when no one had handheld hair dryers at their disposal. It still works and is an excellent way to style hair straight while minimizing damage from heat styling. This makes the doobie especially good for straightening relaxed or chemically processed hair that is fragile. It does, however, require lots of time. You can speed up the drying process by sitting under a hood dryer—the dryer that causes the least amount of heat damage to the hair.

Tools

- **Setting lotion, leave-in conditioner**, or a **straightening balm**, if you will be sitting under a hood dryer.
- **One large, round hair roller.** The width of the roller will depend on the length of your hair. Try to get it as large as possible, unless you have a short- to medium–length hairstyle. In that case, the roller should be large enough to wrap the hair around the roller at least once.
- **Roller clips.**
- **Large, strong bobby pins.**
- **Long-tail comb.**

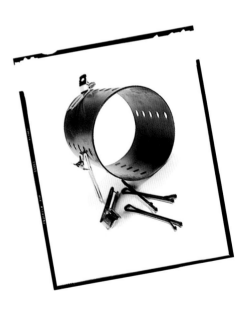

Technique

✔ Start with damp, not soaking wet hair. Prepare the hair with the styling products; use a setting lotion or leave-in conditioner if you will be air-drying, or a straightening balm—most are meant to be used with heat—if you will be sitting under a hood dryer.

✔ At the crown, section the hair off at a width no wider than the roller. If you tend to have dry ends, apply a light extra layer of leave-in conditioner. Comb hair smoothly and hold the section taut, up and away from the scalp.

✔ Place the roller at the tip of the section. Be sure to smooth the ends with your fingertips and continue smoothing the hair as you wrap it around the roller.

✔ Slowly and evenly roll roller and hair down to the scalp.

✔ Secure the roller to the scalp with carefully placed roller clips. Be sure to place the clips close to the roller. Roller clips have a special dent toward the spring that allows them to sit at the edge of the roller without crimping the hair.

✔ Use the long-tail comb to make a part in the hair that remains loose around the back, front, and sides.

✔ Using the comb and your hands, comb, wrap, and press the hair, laying it flat in a giant swirl around your scalp.

✔ With large bobby pins, secure the hair flat against the head as you go around. Place a bobby pin every two inches or so to secure hair as you work, eventually wrapping all the remaining hair around your head. If you have very long hair, your wrap may overlap.

✔ When your hair is nearly dry, remove the pins from the hair wrapped around the front and the sides. Rewrap hair in the opposite direction.

✔ Remove the doobie when hair is absolutely bone-dry.

✔ Use a hair dryer and brush to lightly style the hair, going over any spots the bobby pins may have dented.

✔ As you would after having blow-dried the hair, lightly apply pomade, silicon or hairdressing cream to the ends to keep them soft and prevent frizzing.

Some Latinas leave their doobies for the weekend, when they can wrap their hair in the morning and spend the rest of the day doing chores or getting work done at home. Others use the doobie to wrap their dry, already-straightened hair at night. This allows the straight style to last throughout the week.

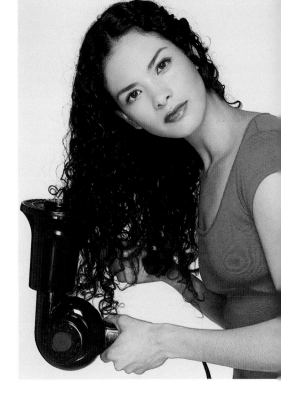

Diffuser attachments can be bought separately.

Blow-drying hair curly

Whether your curls are natural or you have a perm, certain styling techniques and products can help ensure that your curls stay curls instead of turning into frizz.

Tools

- **Hair dryer with diffuser attachment.**
- **Light, spray leave-in conditioner.**

Technique

✔ Apply leave-in conditioner after washing. Allow hair to air-dry for about 10 minutes. Then, tilting the head down, flip the hair forward and blow-dry hair near the scalp with a diffuser. When this area is fairly dry, gently flip hair back and allow the rest to dry naturally. For maximum volume, when hair is completely dry, scrunch it with fingers, doing so with product if you want extra curls. Never disturb hair while it is in the process of drying. The result will be perfect, intact curls.

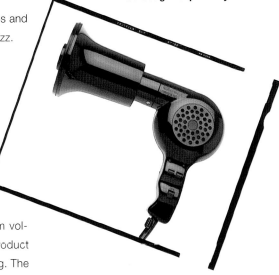

✔ If you don't want annoying baby hairs to curl up tightly around your hairline, creating a tiny fuzz, place a large terry cloth headband at the hairline as your hair dries. If you want the hair around your hairline to dry off of your face, use butterfly clips along the hairline to lift the hair up and away from your face as it dries.

Getting the Right **Chemistry**

IN ADDITION TO BEING GIVEN A FABULOUS RANGE OF HAIR TEXTURES and colors due to our genes, science and chemistry have allowed us to experiment with all kinds of changes to our hair. The one thing you should learn from this chapter, however: Chemically treated hair is high-maintenance hair. It requires special treatment that needs to be consistent in order for the hair health to be maintained.

When you determine what process is right for your hair type, or the style you are trying to achieve, you then have to build your hair-care routine around the treatments you subject it to. A chemical process alone doesn't make beautiful hair—it's the process paired with the right hair-care regimen that is the real secret.

Before undergoing any chemical treatment, be it color or perm or relaxer, there are a few things to keep in mind:

• Be absolutely honest with your stylist about what's been done to your hair before. Previous treatments affect not only the health of your hair but also how your hair responds to a new process. Apprise your hairdresser of anything you have done to your hair during the past two years. The longer your hair, the more likely it still bears the effects of those treatments. Henna, for example, adds a coating to the hair, so getting a perm is more difficult since the extent to which the hair will absorb the chemicals is limited.

• A good hairstylist will give you a thorough consultation before any chemical treatment is done. One of the main objectives of a consultation is for the hairstylist to assess your hair's overall health. If your hair is damaged, or you are growing out a prior chemical treatment, your stylist may suggest waiting a few months or undergoing regular deep-conditioning regimens to return your hair to a healthier state before proceeding with a new treatment. If that is the case, take the advice and wait until your hair is healthy before getting the procedure.

• The stylist will also assess your hair type. Hair type generally refers to the thickness, hydration level, and texture of your natural hair, and whether or not you have gray hair. These elements should all be taken into consideration before going ahead with any chemical treatments that will alter the texture or color of your hair, since certain types may be resistant to texture or color changes.

Did you know? Latinas are twice as likely as non-Hispanic women to have spent $200 or more on hair care in the last six months.

Healthy hair, regardless of texture or color, is beautiful hair.

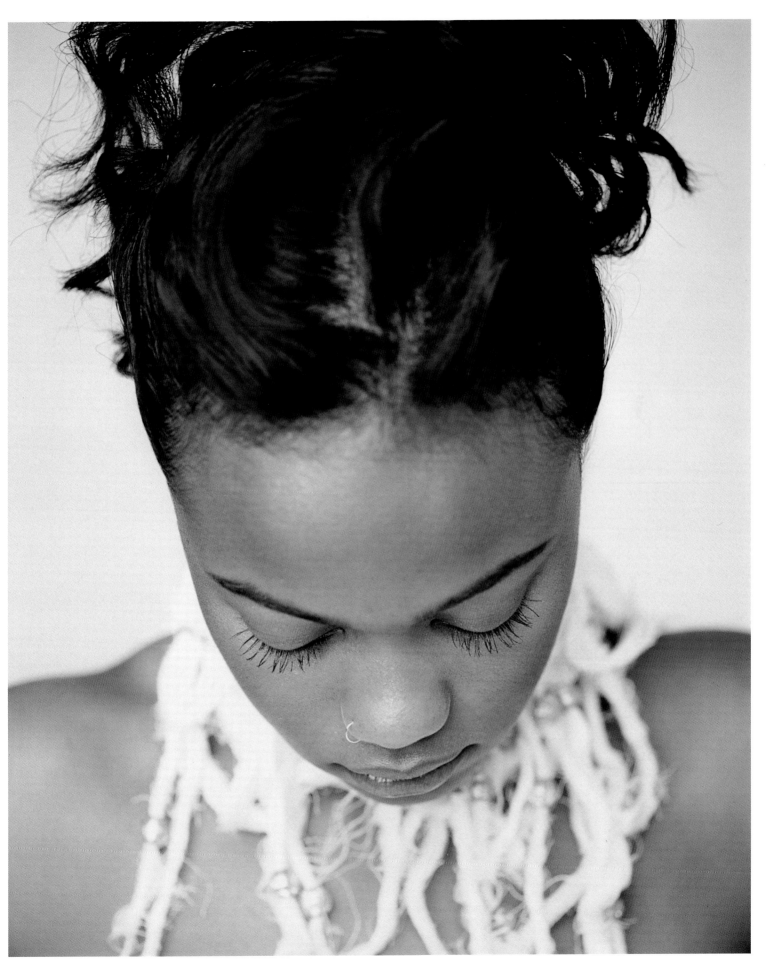

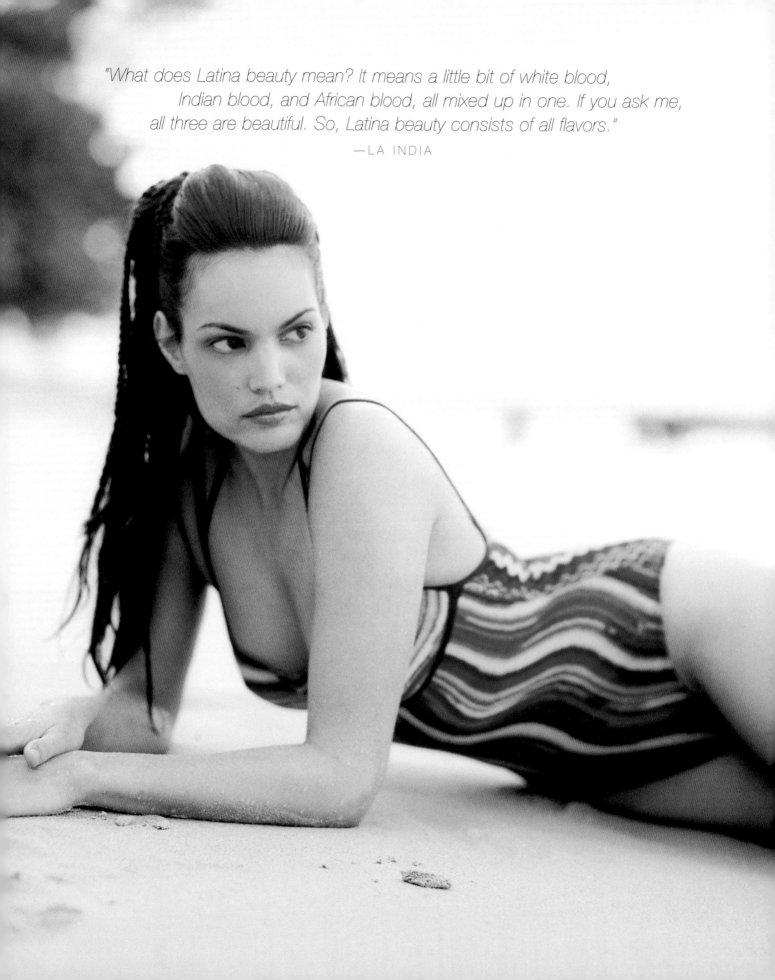

"What does Latina beauty mean? It means a little bit of white blood,
            Indian blood, and African blood, all mixed up in one. If you ask me,
            all three are beautiful. So, Latina beauty consists of all flavors."
                                            —LA INDIA

- Review what follow-up treatments you will need to undergo after the procedure. Changes may include a new shampoo and conditioner for permed or colored hair. Also, hair loses nutrients after a perm, so ask your stylist about conditioning treatments required to return the hair to its optimal, healthy state.
- Always do a strand test before chemically treating hair. You can do it at home or have the hairdresser do it. Remove a strand of hair from your head. Pull on it from both ends. If the hair breaks easily, it has little elasticity and any chemical work will cause it to break further.
- Talk to your hairdresser about special circumstances that need to be taken into consideration. Salt water, for example, tends to revert relaxed hair, and a sun-drenched week at the beach can change the hair color you just spent a fortune on at the salon. A good hairstylist will tell you how to deal with these changes and the necessary precautions to take.
- The frequency with which you wash your hair may have to change after any chemical treatment is done. Shampooing relaxed, permed, or colored hair strips it of protective oils and moisture. Unless you have extremely fine, thin hair that is also very oily, chemically treated hair should be washed no more than every three to four days.
- Conversely, the amount of conditioning you do to your hair may have to increase. Conditioning the hair every day, either through the frequent application of a leave-in conditioner or by using hairdressing creams and moisturizing products during styling, may be recommended. Even *hermanas* who have fine, oily hair that is colored or permed may need extra conditioning on the ends.
- Tell your hairdresser if you are taking birth-control pills, because they can affect chemical treatments.
- Definitely tell your hairdresser if you are pregnant and intend to breastfeed.

Changing texture: Going curly or straight

With the exception of temporary body waves, all textural changes to hair, whether straightening or curling, are permanent, which is to say the effects won't disappear completely until you cut them off. And be forewarned that allowing too much time between touch-ups can lead to hair breakage, since the lack of uniformity weakens the shaft. Whether you want to go curly or straight, know when you do it that you will be living with the results for some time.

Beauty myth busted!

Mami **says:** "Don't use other people's brushes. You'll get dandruff."

Doctor says: "Dandruff is a common condition of the scalp and is not contagious"—that from Los Angeles–based physician John J. Estrada, M.D. While its exact cause is unclear, dandruff is simply an excess shedding of the skin, Dr. Estrada explains. Some people with the condition have overactive oil-production glands, others elevated levels of naturally present fungus and bacteria. Possible contributors include heredity, food allergies, excessive sweating, yeast infections, alkaline soaps, and stress.

Multitextured hair

SOME WOMEN NATURALLY HAVE MORE THAN ONE TEXTURE TO THEIR HAIR. NELSON BARRETO OF New York City's Ene Hair Salon suggests you speak to your stylist about the best way to deal with combination hair, or hair that is both curly and straight. Options include giving a curly perm to the straight sections or to relax the curly sections. Either choice will affect how much time you spend styling your hair as well as the hair care regimen, so be sure to think about it before deciding.

Changing texture

Process: Texturizer

Description: This process applies a relaxer for a brief period of time in order to loosen the natural curl.

Hair type(s) it's best for: Tightly curled hair.

Touch-up time: Every six to eight weeks. Touch-ups on roots only.

Damage level: Mildest form of a relaxer, so the damage to healthy hair is minimal.

Hair-care adjustment: Leave-in conditioner and moisturizing products should be incorporated into hair-care regimen. Since you will have the option of styling hair straight or curly, use styling products specific to each look.

Relaxed hair tips

SANTA CRUZ, WHO OWNS A SALON IN NEW York City and caters to the tresses of actress Lauren Velez, suggests the following tips for relaxed hair:

• If you have a normal-to-dry scalp, sleep on a silk pillowcase. Cotton pillowcases soak up the natural oils of the hair, which are protective and beneficial to relaxed hair. Cotton pillowcases also have less "slide" and can cause hair to break as you sleep.

• If you have an oily scalp, switch to a cotton pillowcase. If the scalp is oily but hair is dry at the ends because of chemical treating, part the hair and put it up into two ponytails. This allows the oils in the scalp and around the hairline to be absorbed by the cotton pillowcase

• Use leave-in conditioner religiously. The light spray-on ones are best for frequent use, especially if you have very thin hair.

• Do a deep-conditioning protein treatment every two weeks.

• Shampoo and condition the hair every four to six days. Once every five days is optimal. If you go to the gym and perspire a lot, wash every four days. If you are in an environment where there is a lot of smoke, you may need to shampoo every three to four days.

• If you comb or brush your hair, don't start at the top of the head and pull the comb or brush through—that will break it. Start at the ends and gradually work your way up to the top in small portions.

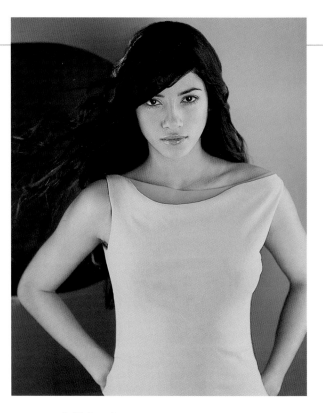

Process: Mild relaxer

Description: A relaxer for the hair with more oil and conditioning agents, to control level and speed of activation. A mild relaxer will loosen a curl or, on some hair, cause it to go straight.

Hair type(s) it's best for: Fine hair with a looser curl.

Touch-up time: Every six to eight weeks. Touch-ups on roots only.

Damage level: Slightly harsher than a texturizer, so you may notice more dryness.

Hair-care adjustment: Select shampoo and conditioner for chemically treated hair. Use leave-in conditioner and moisturizing products to style and protect. If hair is normally dry, regular monthly deep-conditioning treatments are recommended.

Process: Regular relaxer

Description: Stronger than the mild relaxer, it also works faster.

Hair type(s) it's best for: Slightly thicker hair with a tighter curl.

Touch-up time: Every six to eight weeks. Touch-ups on roots only.

Damage level: Since the product is stronger, it can leave hair quite dehydrated.

Hair-care adjustment: In addition to shampoo and conditioner for chemically treated hair, and moisturizing products to style and protect, a deep-conditioning protein-replenishing treatment must be incorporated into the hair-care routine on a monthly or weekly basis.

Process: Strong relaxer

Description: The most potent relaxer.

Hair type(s) it's best for: Coarse, very tightly curled hair.

Touch-up time: Every six to eight weeks. Touch-ups on roots only.

Damage level: Can be the most damaging if not monitored properly during application; may cause hair to break if left on longer than necessary.

Hair-care adjustment: Return to salon for follow-up moisturizing and protein treatments. Select shampoo and conditioner for chemically treated hair. Use moisturizing products to style and protect and heat-protective styling products when applicable. After the salon treatments have been administered, a deep-conditioning treatment must be incorporated into the hair-care routine.

Process: Dry curl

Description: Body waves for very tightly curled hair. The procedure is essentially a relaxer, followed by a body wave to give a more relaxed curl.

Hair type(s) it's best for: Very curly, kinky hair.

Touch-up time: Every six to eight weeks. Touch-ups on roots only.

Damage level: Very high, because it is double-processed hair. You must commit to laying off the blow-dryer and sticking with the new, looser curls.

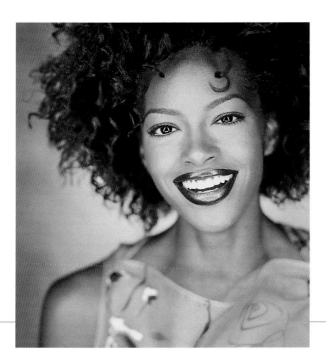

Curly-permed hair tips

- Use a diffuser to blow-dry the hair. As the name implies, these attachments disperse the air as it blows onto the hair, leaving the curl undisturbed.
- Don't use hot water to wash the hair, use warm water. Hot water tends to release whatever effect the perm has on the hair.
- Don't use brushes, only wide-tooth combs.
- If you want to comb permed hair, the time to do it is when you have conditioner in your hair. After that, towel-dry gently and leave it alone.
- Permed hair is fragile and prone to breakage. Don't use rubber bands to tie the hair back or anything that has a tight grip and can pull hair out. Use bands covered in fabric if you want to pull it back.

Hair-care adjustment: Return to salon for follow-up moisturizing and protein treatments. Use a very gentle, ultra-moisturizing shampoo and conditioner. A deep-conditioning treatment must be incorporated into the hair-care routine.

Process: Permanent wave

Description: Gives curls to straight hair. Degree and type of curl depends on the size and type of rod and the way the curl is rolled.

Touch-up time: Every six to eight weeks. Touch-ups on roots only.

Damage level: Can be high.

Hair-care adjustment: Perms dry out the hair considerably. Use a leave-in conditioner in a spray form to protect hair without weighing down curls. Use deep-conditioning treatment to replace lost moisture and protein on a weekly or monthly basis, depending on the condition of your hair.

Process: Semi-permanent wave

Description: This process works similarly to semi-permanent hair color in that the solution does not penetrate the hair shaft completely. A semi-permanent wave gives a light body boost to hair.

Touch-up time: After five to ten washings.

Damage level: Light, since it doesn't radically penetrate the hair or change its composition. Check with your stylist, though, before experimenting with this process on colored hair.

Hair-care adjustment: None, since the effects go away rather quickly.

Changing hair color

Process: Henna

Description: An organic hair dye derived from plants, it enriches the depth of your own color.

Hair type(s) it's best for: Hair that is nonfrizzy and "virgin" (untouched by chemical processes).

Touch-up time: Retouch every four to six weeks. The color lasts until it is cut off. Henna makes hair resistant to other chemical treatments, which means you can't try to color over the henna with regular coloring agents.

Damage level: Coats hair shaft and does not allow it to breathe, which can cause hair to loose elasticity.

Hair-care adjustment: Since henna makes hair prone to snapping and breaking, style with care and keep well moisturized.

Process: Semi-permanent color

Definition: Coats the hair, depositing color without completely opening the hair cuticle.

Hair type(s) it's best for: Excellent for fine hair because it only deposits color and gives hair more body. Best option for permed hair, since it is less damaging than permanent color.

Touch-up time: Approximately four to six shampoos.

Damage level: Has no ammonia or peroxide, so no damage to hair.

Hair-care adjustment: Color-enhancing shampoos can help the color last, but this is not recommended for women who have both color and a perm; they would be better served with a moisturizing shampoo and conditioner.

Process: Demi-permanent color

Description: Ammonia-based color mixed with low amounts of peroxide. Cannot dramatically lighten hair color.

Hair type(s) it's best for: Can be used in conjunction with other chemical procedures such as relaxers or perms, but you must wait at least two weeks between procedures. Also good for covering gray, especially if hair has also been relaxed or permed.

Touch-up time: Approximately 24 shampoos.

Damage level: Minimal damage to hair if it is only color, more if hair must be stripped first (see Blonding).

Hair-care adjustment: Use shampoos for color-treated hair and leave-in conditioner; condition every time you wash. If you heat-style your hair, include a regular deep-conditioning treatment in your regimen one to two times per month.

Process: Permanent color

Description: Deposits pigment in hair shaft, penetrating hair cuticle. The only option for dramatically changing hair color; necessary if you want to go blond.

Hair type(s) it's best for: Hair that has no other chemical processes in it. This is the process that most effectively covers gray hair. If you have a perm, permanent color can be done, but it must be done with caution. It's also a good option for fine, thin hair, since the procedure lifts the hair cuticle, expanding the hair and making it easier to style.

Touch-up time: Retouch every four to six weeks. The color lasts until it is cut off.

Damage level: More damage is done if hair must be stripped first (see Blonding).

Hair-care adjustment: Use gentle, moisturizing shampoos and conditioners for color-treated hair. Condition every time you wash. If you also heat-style your hair, incorporate a regular deep-conditioning treatment into your regimen two to three times a month.

Process: Highlights

Description: Hair strands are stripped of natural color. Can be an effective alternative to overall blonding, or a

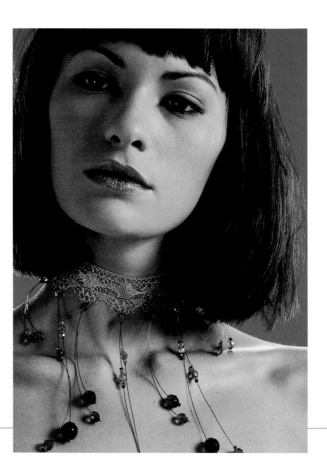

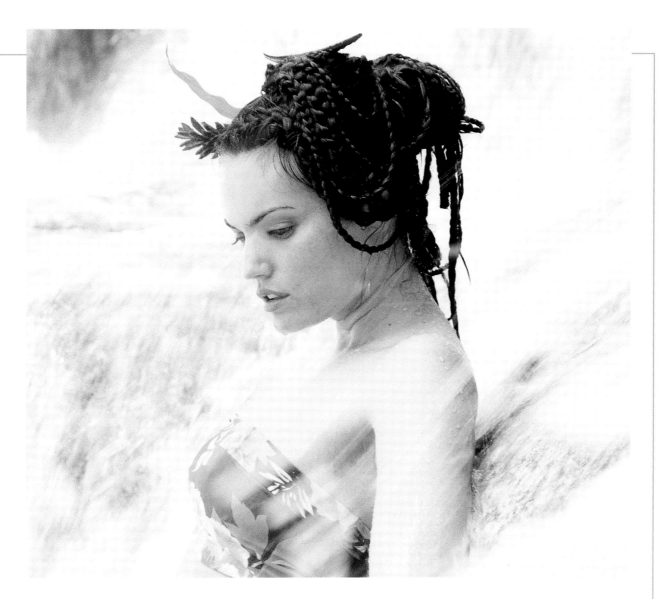

blending, minimizing method for gray hair. Permanent hair color is applied in certain areas all over the hair using different techniques.

Hair type(s) it's best for: Can be done on hair that has been chemically treated, but the hair must be healthy and well conditioned.

Touch-up time: Touch-ups can stretch from two to three months, since the roots are less obvious.

Damage level: Depends on what types of highlights are done. Those with peroxide or ammonia in the formula are harsher.

Hair-care adjustment: Dryness may be noticeable on highlighted parts. Use moisturizing hairdressing cream on those areas or on ends.

Process: Blonding

Description: Natural hair color is stripped away using peroxide. A permanent, lighter hair color is then applied to replace it.

Hair type(s) it's best for: Natural, healthy hair that has had no other chemical treatments. It can be used on permed hair, but most hairstylists advise against it.

Touch-up time: Until it grows or is cut out. Touch-ups should be done every four to six weeks on roots only.

Damage level: Very high. This is double-processed hair.

Hair-care adjustment: Return to salon for follow-up moisturizing and protein treatments. In addition to the appropriate moisturizing products, a deep-conditioning treatment must be incorporated into the regular hair-care routine.

Did you **know?** | **Latinas are 41 percent more likely than non-Hispanic women to color their hair at home.**

Making **the Cut**

WHAT MAKES A GREAT HAIRCUT? A HAIRSTYLIST WILL TAKE INTO account the following factors:

• **Your lifestyle.** Do you have three kids and only twenty minutes to shower and get ready in the morning? Do you work out every other day? Do you need versatile hair that can be pulled back for the weekend, but also styled conservatively for your work environment? A great cut will complement, not compete with, your lifestyle.

• **The time you are willing to spend on it.** This seems like a lifestyle question, but it's really one of personal commitment. We all know at least one Latina who holds down a demanding job, has a house and kids, and still finds time to make it to the hairdresser once a week for her deep-conditioning treatment and weekly styling. For her, the issue is simple: Her hair is important, and she will find the time. Be honest with yourself when it comes to discussing this with your stylist.

• **Your hair texture.** This dovetails with the time issue. If your hair is an explosion of curls and you bring your hairdresser a photo of Jennifer Lopez during her blonde ambition, swingy-straight incarnation, be honest: Are you willing to spend a twice-weekly, hour-long session under the dryer and with the straightening iron to get that look?

• **The shape of your face.** Even though it seems old-fashioned and limiting to suggest that certain face shapes should get certain styles, the reality of the situation is that if you want you hair to draw attention to certain features (say, your eyes) and detract from other areas (like the roundness of your face), some styles are more flattering than others. Highlights in the hair can also be used effectively for the same purpose.

• **Your height.** How long is too long? Generally, anything past your bra line is too long. It weighs the hair down and makes it look flat. If you have very curly hair, a bit of length weighs the hair, keeping it curly and beautiful. If you are short, long hair can overwhelm you, making you appear even shorter. Long hair also tends to lie very flat on the top of the head, which makes your face look more circular if it is round to begin with.

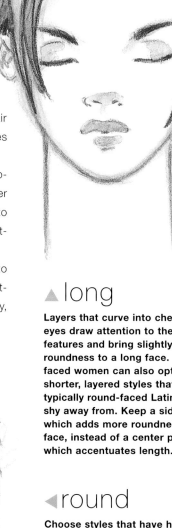

▲long

Layers that curve into cheeks and eyes draw attention to these features and bring slightly more roundness to a long face. Long-faced women can also opt for the shorter, layered styles that typically round-faced Latinas may shy away from. Keep a side part, which adds more roundness to the face, instead of a center part, which accentuates length.

◀round

Choose styles that have height at the crown, helping to elongate the face. If you have long hair, updo *moños*, while not necessarily appropriate for everyday wear, have a lengthening effect as well. Avoid bangs, which cut the face in half, leaving it even more round- and youthful-looking. Another option: Get highlights at the crown of the head. Light hair at the crown also gives the appearance of height at the top of the head.

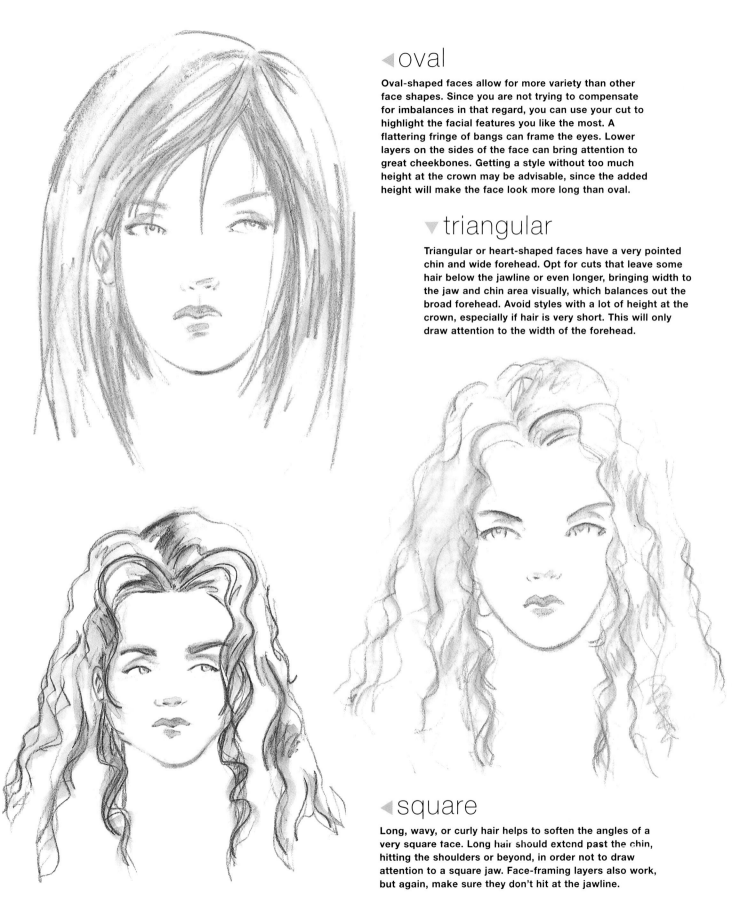

◀ oval

Oval-shaped faces allow for more variety than other face shapes. Since you are not trying to compensate for imbalances in that regard, you can use your cut to highlight the facial features you like the most. A flattering fringe of bangs can frame the eyes. Lower layers on the sides of the face can bring attention to great cheekbones. Getting a style without too much height at the crown may be advisable, since the added height will make the face look more long than oval.

▼ triangular

Triangular or heart-shaped faces have a very pointed chin and wide forehead. Opt for cuts that leave some hair below the jawline or even longer, bringing width to the jaw and chin area visually, which balances out the broad forehead. Avoid styles with a lot of height at the crown, especially if hair is very short. This will only draw attention to the width of the forehead.

◀ square

Long, wavy, or curly hair helps to soften the angles of a very square face. Long hair should extend past the chin, hitting the shoulders or beyond, in order not to draw attention to a square jaw. Face-framing layers also work, but again, make sure they don't hit at the jawline.

"Of course it's my hair, I paid for it!"
Your Guide to Faking It

Wigs

WIGS MAKE THE BOLDEST STATEMENT OF ALL AND CAN REALLY CHANGE your whole look. Experiment not only with length and texture changes, but color changes as well. Since hair color has such an impact, you might find that you will want to adjust your makeup colors to suit the new look as well. Unless you will be wearing it every day, skip the expense of human hair and go for a synthetic wig. Wigs come in sizes, and it's important to take the time to get the right fit.

Extensions

Jennifer Lopez, Salma Hayek, and Patricia Velasquez have all used extensions to change their look. Extensions can be done in various ways. Select your method and hair type (synthetic or human) based on how much you are willing to spend and how long you want the extensions to last. Hair can be purchased at beauty supply stores. If you are going to a salon to do this, check with your stylist about whether you should buy the hair first and what method they recommend. Some stylists recommend certain methods of application over others.

• **Bonding.** This process involves taking very small sections of your hair and "bonding" bundles of hair onto your own at the root with a special wax-based glue that fuses yours and the artificial hair. You do need to use a special comb for bonded hair, but beyond that it can be washed and styled as usual. A special remover is needed to dissolve the wax-based glue and take off the extensions. Done properly, this method can last up to three months. Because of the longevity, it is best to get human hair in a color that complements your own.

• **Gluing.** A more temporary method—it lasts as long as you can stand not to wash your hair—this option requires that you glue lengths of extensions directly onto your scalp. Careful placement at the sides and back and even around the

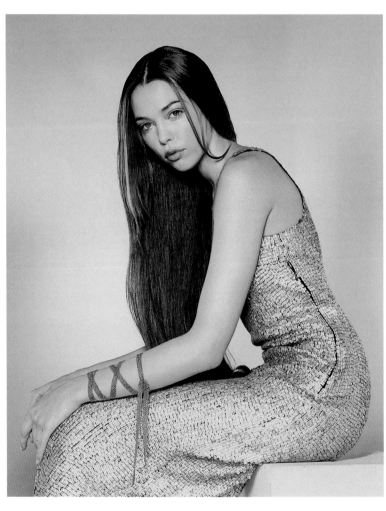

Extensions add length and drama.

Opposite: This model's real hair goes past her shoulders. Here, she wears a wig that was cut to create a choppy, sexy new look.

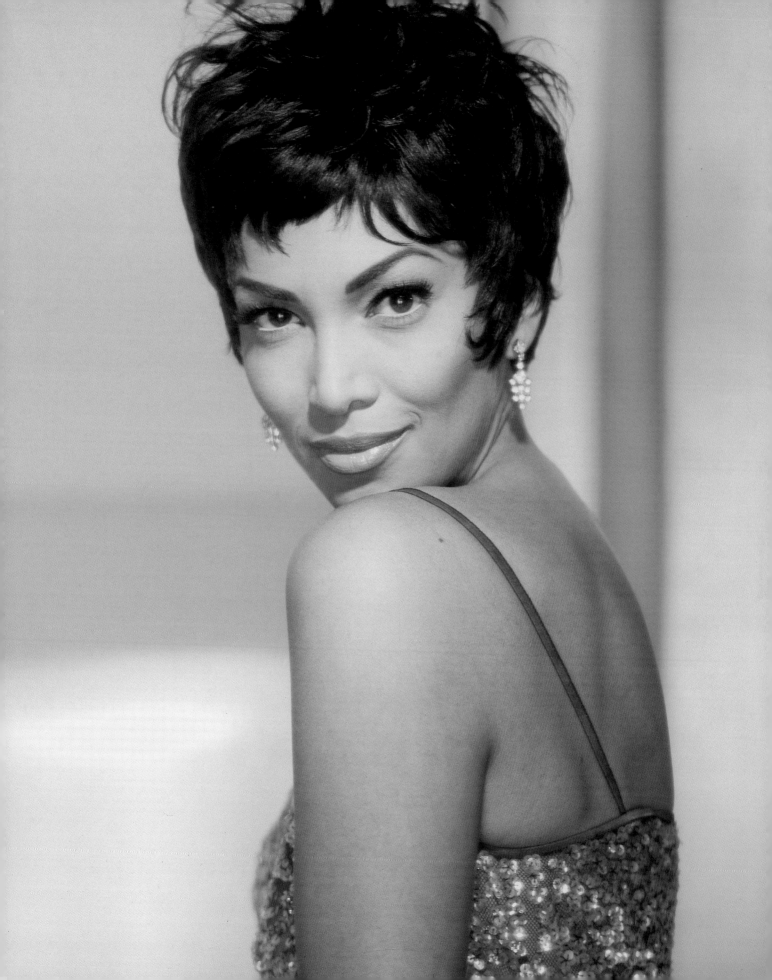

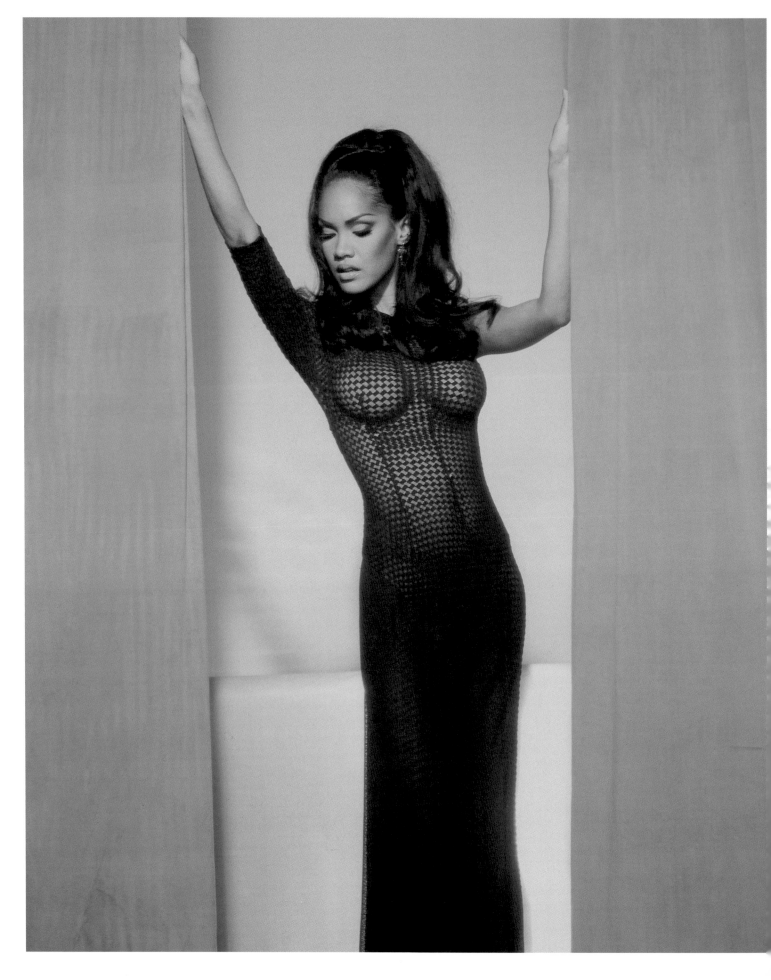

crown make it effective for adding new length and color to your hair. Due to the procedure's temporary nature, artificial hair makes more sense. A special glue remover is required to take out the extensions.

• **Clips.** The best option for a fun night out. Small wefts of hair are secured in your hair near the scalp using clips with teeth that anchor the extensions to the shaft. The wefts of hair are very small, so they can be placed almost anywhere on the head, as long as you are careful to blend it with your natural hair. Since it's so temporary, have fun by experimenting with color and texture.

• **Braiding.** Extensions can also be braided into the hair. Tiny sections of your hair (usually at the back and the sides, where your natural hair can conceal the braids) are used to braid in sections of extensions. The braid is then sewn with special thread to secure the hair to yours. Braiding, like bonding, lasts up to three months.

Other types of braid extensions begin at the scalp and are placed all over the head. These can be an excellent option for growing out hair that has been relaxed, since the mixed texture (relaxed and natural) can make the hair prone to breakage. Braid-sheen oil keeps braids shiny and healthy.

Falls

These sections of hair attached to a base work like half-wigs. The placement of the base on the head, as well as the length of the fall, are what determine the look. Falls are mostly used for adding length or fullness, making them the best options for evenings or special occasions. Again, since it will probably only be used occasionally, go for synthetic over human hair. Most falls come with comb attachments, but you will probably need to anchor the piece more securely with additional bobby pins.

Weave

This is an all-day process that can completely change your look. A stylist braids your entire head (with the exception of hair along the hairline, which is left alone so the weave can blend) into a cornrow. Hair is then sewn onto the cornrow. Removal of the weave involves simply cutting the strings that were sewn.

Weaves are expensive, and with good reason: The labor involved is intensive, and the hair used should be human hair. Purchase hair in a texture that matches how you will be wearing yours, in a color that will blend at the hairline.

Opposite: A fall gave this model's hair height, creating a retro style reminiscent of the '60s.

Tool time: Caring for hair implements

GOOD HAIR TOOLS CAN BE EXPENSIVE, BUT are worth the cost. They also demand a certain amount of maintenance. It is time well spent. Maricela Marquez, a master hairstylist at Sergio's in San Antonio, Texas, has these tips for tool upkeep:

• **Brushes.** Remove old hair from the brush using a towel to grab it or a long-tail teasing comb to lift the hair vertically off the brush. To remove dirt and oil that may still cling to the bristles after hair has been removed, place brushes in a sinkful of warm water and diluted shampoo or antibacterial dishwashing liquid.

• **Flatirons/curling irons.** Both types of irons can acquire buildup if you use product in the hair. Plug in the iron and put it on high heat. Using a clean rag folded up several times, apply oven cleaner to dissolve the film.

• **Blow-dryer.** Professional dryers usually have a screen in the back of the dryer that you can remove in order to clean out lint. If lint accumulates, the dryer's "motor" will be less effective. If your dryer does not have a removable screen, use tweezers to lift lint from the screen.

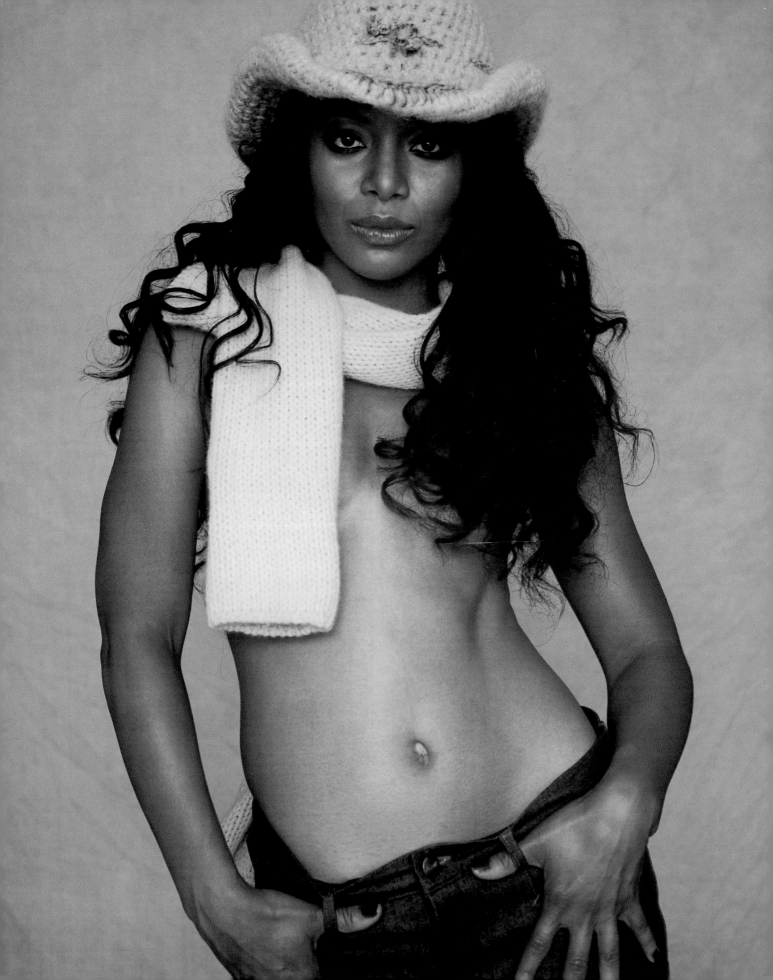

Get the Glow:
Sensual, Smooth Skin

YOUR SKIN, LIKE YOUR HAIR AND YOUR BODY, CHANGES. IT FLUCTUATES DUE TO INTERNAL factors, like the time of the month and your age, and to external factors, such as the time of year, the climate you are in, and lifestyle choices—how much you smoke or drink, say, or how much time you spend in the sun without sun protection. Understanding this essential fact of life will help make your skin-care choices much easier. When you approach it as a process that requires fluidity with distinct solutions at different times of the year, your ability to keep your skin looking its best is maximized.

While your skin probably stays true to one basic skin type throughout the year, you may find that the same routine all of a sudden does not produce the results it did in the past. This is when you need to adapt your routine. Building the basic elements of a good skin-care pattern, then knowing when and what to adapt and change is the best defense.

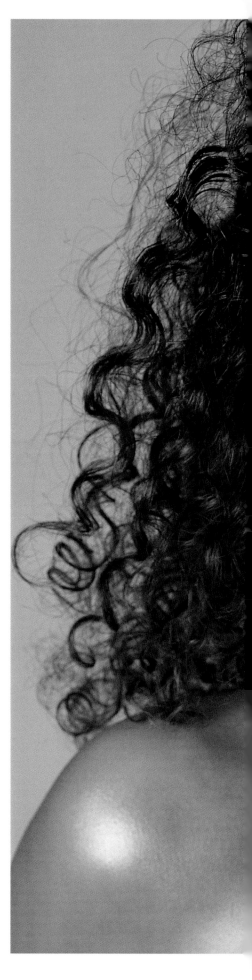

"I think physical beauty in a woman is really clean skin and bright eyes and then whatever you put on top of that — whether you choose to put makeup on it or moisturizer or a little base. It's health and vibrancy that makes one beautiful."

— ELIZABETH PEÑA

Basic **Face**

¿Cual es tu tipo?

To determine your skin type, do the tissue test:

✔ Wash your face.

✔ Wait 15 minutes, then blot your face with a tissue or oil-blotting paper.

● If the tissue has oily spots on it, you have oily skin.

● If the tissue only picks up oil after it is pressed to the T-zone area (forehead, nose, and chin), you have combination skin.

● If you have very few blotches on the tissue, you have normal skin.

● If the tissue is completely free of blotches, you have dry skin.

Most women need certain staples in their skin-care routines. The products you select should depend on your skin type.

Dry Skin

Dry skin is characterized by very small pores. Prone to flakiness, dry skin can also be sensitive.

Oily Skin

Large pores, especially on the nose, forehead, or even on the back and chest, are one of the primary characteristics of oily skin. Oily skin is caused by increased secretion from the sebaceous (oil-producing) glands in the hair follicles. Oil glands are controlled by hormones, which is one of the reasons that birth-control pills are useful in controlling acne. Latinas, and women of color in general, tend to have oilier skin than Caucasian women.

Combination

A lot of people fall into this category, which essentially means that you have an oily T-zone and dry cheeks. With this skin type, where you apply skin-care products is as important as what type you use.

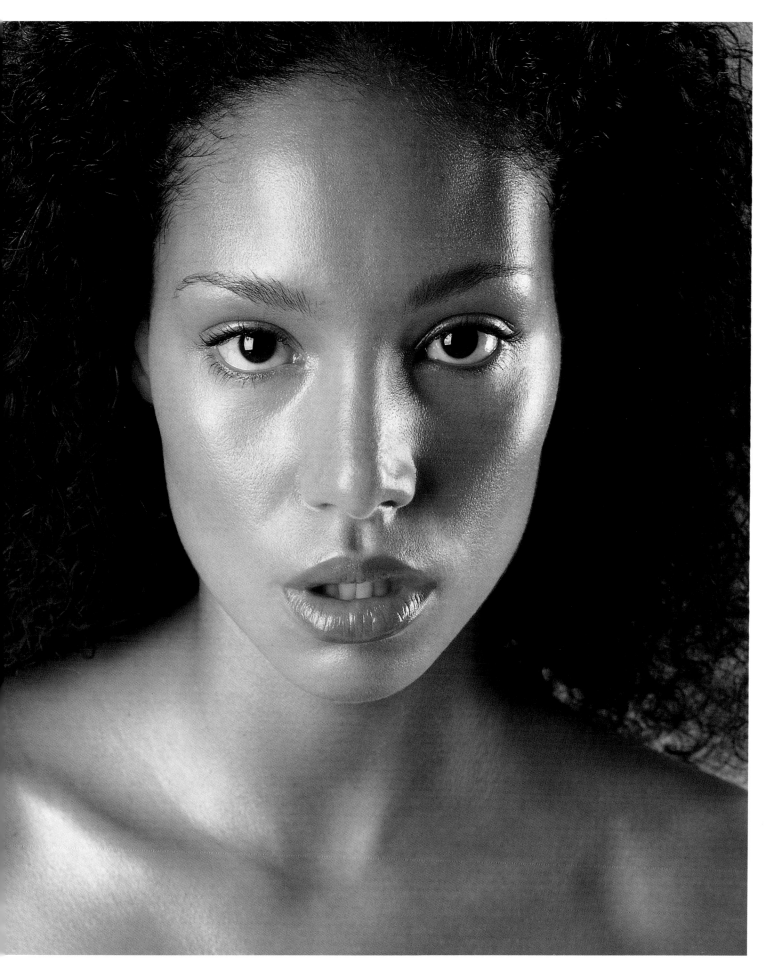

What You **Absolutely** Need

EVERY WOMAN SHOULD INCLUDE THESE BASIC ELEMENTS IN HER skin-care routine:

Cleanser

The most important selection for good skin care. A little guided experimentation and the willingness to invest some money and time is necessary. Once you find something that works for you, stick with it.

So many cleansers on the market right now do so many things in addition to just cleaning—from controlling excess oil to exfoliating skin to moisturizing. These extras are nice if they work, but the priority in any cleanser should be that it cleanses without stripping or drying the skin's surface. Your face should feel soft, pliable, and pampered. If your skin feels tight after cleansing, you need to switch to a cleanser that is not so harsh.

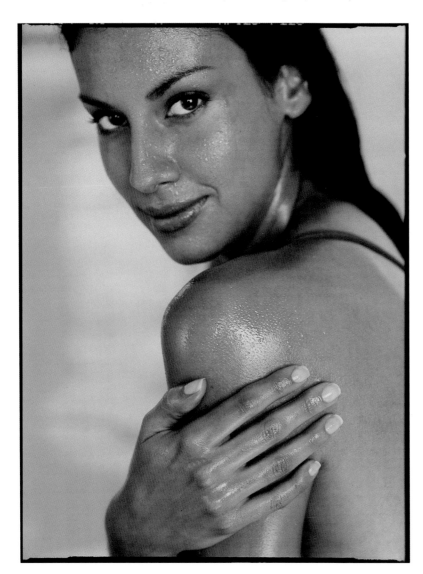

- **Oily or acne-prone.** Look for cleansers in the form of gels or bars.
- **Dry skin.** Experiment with cream-based or creamy cleansers.
- **Combination skin.** Take your pick of the type, but don't use a product that is specifically for one type of skin or the other. Look for cleansers for "normal" or combination skin.

Sun protection

Wearing hats, sunglasses, and a sunscreen with a sun protection factor (SPF) of 15 or higher is the only way to prevent the premature wrinkles and *manchas* that are the result of sun damage. A lot of Latinas think that a daily suncscreen is for white women or *güeras*. "We get beautiful and brown," we tell ourselves. Similarly, we commonly believe that skin cancer is only a Caucasian concern.

Regardless of how brown and beautiful you are, you need to make the application of sunscreen a central, daily part of your skin-care routine. A broad-spectrum SPF formula protects you from both UVA and UVB rays. UVA, known as the "aging" rays

Dicho y hecho

WONDERING WHICH INGREDIENTS DO WHAT FOR your skin? Here is the info, as well as other buzzwords you need to know when you buy skin-care products.

Free radicals: A by-product of UV rays, smoke, and pollution, free radicals are unstable molecules that damage skin cells and speed aging of skin.

Anti-oxidants: Vitamins A, C, and E and chemicals called polyphenols that, applied topically, prevent or reduce the destructive effects of free radicals.

Vitamin A: An antioxidant that enhances the complexion by reducing fine lines and wrinkles.

Vitamin C: An antioxidant that has been shown to prevent wrinkles and skin cancers.

Vitamin E: Another antioxidant that may help protect skin against ultraviolet rays and other free-radical penetration. No hard medical evidence documents its efficacy for external use—but this doesn't stop many Latinas, like the singer La India, from swearing by the benefits of breaking open a capsule and applying its contents to the skin.

Tretinoin: A vitamin A derivative used to unblock pores and reduce sun damage. It is found in prescription medications like Retin-A, Renova, and Avita. Originally used to treat acne, this product became popular among young and old alike when it was found to reduce the appearance of wrinkles.

Retinol: An over-the-counter vitamin A-based product that encourages exfoliation and normalizes the cells lining the pores, so pores don't get blocked below the surface. Skin-care products that contain at least 3 percent retinol can be effective, although not as effective as the prescription vitamin A product Retin-A.

Alpha Hydroxy Acids (AHAs): Often called fruit acids because many are derived from fruit plants, AHAs act as exfoliants to smooth and clear skin. Although they may initially cause a few dry flakes on the skin, with regular long-term use they can help reverse sun damage in the skin's top layer while stimulating collagen and elastin growth in the deeper layers. Common AHAs: glycolic and citric acids.

Beta Hydroxy Acids (BHAs): Milder exfoliants than AHAs, BHAs are also naturally occurring acids primarily derived from plant sources. While some dermatologists claim BHAs are more gentle, they lack the anti-aging and anti–sun damaging properties of AHAs. Common BHAs: salicylic and benzoic acids.

Ceramide: A lipid present in the outer layer of the skin that helps retain moisture. Creams with ceramides in the formula are of benefit to dry, older, or sun-damaged skin that requires more moisture.

Collagen: Protein that maintains the skin's strength, firmness, and fullness. It also helps repair injured skin by building scar tissue. Creams that contain collagen may be good moisturizers, but they don't actually affect the skin's own collagen production.

Elastin: Fibers that give skin its flexibility and elasticity, enabling it to stretch and contract repeatedly with movement. Like collagen, elastin in cream formula might make a good moisturizer, but it can't repair the skin's elastin fibers.

Humectants: Substances that draw water to the skin from the environment or from lower layers of the skin, helping it retain moisture. Common humectants: glycerine, squalene, urea, and sorbitol.

Noncomedogenic or nonacnegenic: These terms refer to products that won't block pores or cause pimples, respectively, but no FDA guidelines govern their labeling. Some products live up to the label, others do not.

Hypo-allergenic: Products less likely to cause an allergic reaction.

Parsol 1789: Also known as avobenzone, this is the only sunblock ingredient besides zinc oxide that the FDA says fully blocks UVA and UVB rays. Parsol 1789 is a chemical sunblock.

Titanium or zinc oxide: Physical sunscreens that form a layer to block the sun's rays from reaching the skin. These appear to cause fewer allergic reactions than chemical sunscreens. Women of color have to make sure that their titanium or zinc oxide formula is micronized in order to avoid the gray or white sheen atop the skin characteristic of earlier forms of sunblock. Darker-skinned Latinas may want to avoid these formulas, since they are still not totally transparent

The following are touted as natural ingredients (few have proven benefits) found in skin-care products:

Grape seed extract: Another antioxidant said to help undo daily damage by free radicals.

Green tea: Rich in the anti-oxidant polyphenolic acid, green tea is a hot new ingredient in skin-care products.

Tea tree oil: A naturally occurring oil with antibacterial and anti-inflammatory properties. The oil itself, however, has been found to block pores, even though it is toted as an acne fighter due to its antibacterial role.

of the sun, are most responsible for deep-tissue damage and premature wrinkling. UVB, the "burning" rays, activate the melanin production of the skin, causing tanning or burning as the immediate outcome. UVB rays are also the cause of skin cancer. *Manchas*, freckles, or age spots are a few less-desirable results of unprotected sun exposure.

Sunscreen comes in two types: physical and chemical blocks. Physical blocks provide a literal shield from the sun's rays. The most common ingredient in physical sunblocks is titanium or zinc oxide (the white cream on a lifeguard's nose). This ingredient was responsible for the pasty, gray look of early SPF formulations, not ground finely enough to prevent the pastiness from being apparent on the skin. Newer formulas, however, are so finely ground that the cream is more transparent and is better absorbed into the skin.

Chemical sunblocks contain ingredients like Parsol 1789 that absorb the harmful rays of the sun. The problem with Parsol 1789, however, is that it loses efficacy after a few hours under the sun, when the chemical compounds that make it effective begin to break down. Right now, Parsol 1789 and zinc oxide are the only two ingredients that are FDA-approved and proven to block both UVA and UVB rays.

When it comes to daily wear SPF formulas, you must consider how the sun protection is delivered. Most zinc oxide-based forms come in a lotion, which can be off-putting for women with oily skin. If you skip an application of moisturizer, however, make sure that the zinc oxide sunscreen is oil-free or a gel-based formula, non-comedogenic, and that the zinc oxide lotion should not cause any extra oiliness or breakouts for women who are prone to acne. Pair it with an oil-free foundation or oil-absorbing powder, and you should be fine. Women with dry skin have their choice of products but may want to consider a sunscreen with moisturizing properties.

As discussed in Chapter 2 ("About Base"), the newest way to get SPF protection is in makeup. This is also a great option for women who feel as if one more layer of product on the face is just too much. Let your skin type be your guide as to which protection you choose. In any case, in whatever form, always use an SPF-formula sunscreen.

Exfoliant

The third element every woman should incorporate into her skin-care routine is some kind of an exfoliant. Exfoliants slough off dead skin cells, giving your skin a fresh appearance, and women of all skin types can benefit from them. For dry skin, exfoliating helps remove ashiness or buildup of dead skin cells that leave the complexion looking dull. For women with oily or acne-prone skin, exfoliation removes the excess dead skin that can clog pores and cause acne. Combination skin reaps double benefits. Those with sensitive skin need not be wary of exfoliants, but more on this below.

As with sunblocks, there are two types of exfoliants: physical and chemical. Physical exfoliants include anything from a washcloth with a slightly rough texture to a facial scrub, to a cream or lotion with tiny granules in the formula that help to remove excess dead skin. Both accomplish the same thing: They remove the dead cells from the top layer of skin. Washcloths are generally used while cleansing the face; facial scrubs can be used in addition to or in place of regular cleanser. Any type of exfoliation should be done gently. Never tug or pull at the skin or scrub roughly. As with cleansing, your skin should feel soft and pampered afterward, not rubbed raw. Exfoliating in this manner should be done up to three times a week. Doing it every day can be excessive and won't really make a difference in the appearance of your skin.

Chemical exfoliants come in the form of lotions or creams or toners that you apply to your face after cleansing. The ingredients in these exfoliants are usually some type of acid: alpha hydroxy (AHA) and beta hydroxy (BHA) acids are the most common. These acids work by gently sloughing off dead cells from the surface of the skin throughout the day. Some of the creams are gentle enough that you can apply them daily, but monitor your skin to see whether that is really necessary. One bonus of AHAs: In cream form—which tends to be slightly more moisturizing, depending on the skin type they are made for—its repairing properties work to minimize wrinkles by ultimately affecting the deeper layers of the skin. Since the top layer of excess skin cells are being removed, fresher, younger skin is being uncovered, diminishing the appearance of fine lines. Chemical exfoliants are not a cure for wrinkles—the best weapon against *arrugas* is and always will be sun protection—but many women who use them notice a nice "plumping" effect on the skin.

As with moisturizers and cleansers, the range of exfoliating creams has broadened beyond the targeted categories of oily, dry, or combination skin. There are exfoliating creams for the hands, undereye area, lips, body, and feet. When it comes to the face, the general rules outlined above are the most helpful: Stick to a formula that matches your skin type.

Sensitive skin types should incorporate exfoliation with a very gentle facial scrub or with a soft washcloth massage. Stay away from chemical exfoliants altogether.

Nice **Extras**

Moisturizer

You may be surprised not to see this included in the "must have" section. A lot of estheticians swear that all skin types, regardless of how oily, need to be moisturized. But dermatologists tell their patients to use it only if they need it. The

A bad acid trip

EXFOLIATING CREAMS ARE NOW MADE WITH different types of acids for different areas of the face and body. A lot of these products can be useful in combating ashiness on the elbows or hands, as well as diminishing hard skin on the feet. But when is it too much?

Most women only need to incorporate one exfoliating step into their routine for each part of their body up to three times a week. Don't double up. If you exfoliate with a loofah in the shower, there is no reason to apply exfoliating body cream.

The face is where women run the most risk of overexfoliation. Many moisturizers, cleansers, facial masks, and spot-treatments for acne have some type of acid in them. The rule with the face, as with the body, is to stick to one product or one regular step, and your skin should be fine. When it comes to blemishes, apply acne medication on areas prone to developing them, but refrain from adding exfoliating creams over that. Too much will leave your skin tight and dry.

Many women who make the mistake of loading up on too many skin-care products with some type of exfoliating chemical in them end up convinced that they have "sensitive" skin, when in fact they are suffering from product overload.

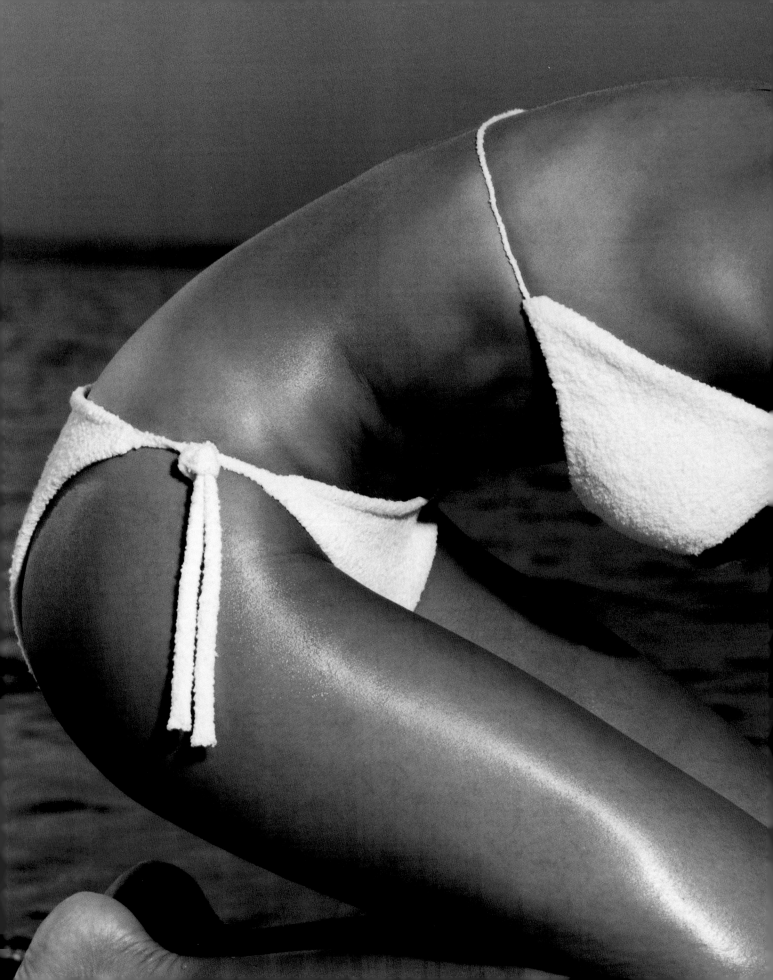

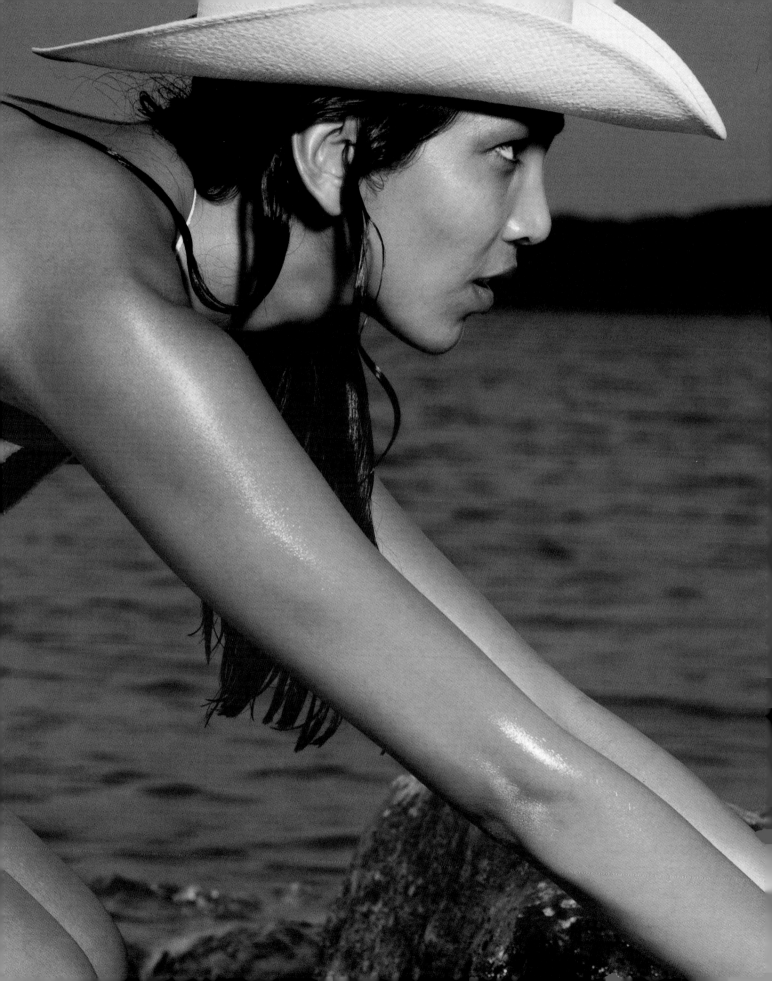

Mami says: "*Para de comer chocolate!* It will give you *espinillas*."

Doctor says: Hershey's kisses, anyone? "Acne has nothing to do with food habits," explains Ana L. Rodriguez, a dermatologist in San Marcos, Texas. When overactive hormones cause the skin to produce excessive sebum, the skin's natural oil, you get clogged pores and oily skin, which leads to acne. Such over-enthusiastic *aceite* output, combined with bacteria that live in the follicles, causes irritation and inflammation. Personal habits can have an effect as well. "Cleaning your skin improperly and applying oily makeup and greasy creams make it worse," Rodriguez says.

confusion evolves around this: Dry skin requires hydration (water) and oil, while oily skin makes too much oil yet still needs to be hydrated. If you have oily skin, an oil-free SPF formula should provide all the hydration required. Women with combination and normal skin should apply moisturizer only where it is needed—usually on the cheeks—and are probably better off with the lighter, oil-free formulas.

If you have dry skin, on the other hand, moisturizer is a step you can't live without. Stick to moisturizers made specifically for your skin type. You can also look into other skin-care products that have moisturizing benefits, like foundations or SPF formulas that moisturize. For Latinas with dry skin and who are prone to acne, select an oil-free moisturizer.

Eye cream

Most women look at this as a necessary skin-care step, especially since eye creams now promise to do everything from reduce puffiness to minimize *patas de gallina* to diminish dark *ojeras*. The bottom line is this: The skin around the eyes is very thin and produces little oil, and since the eyes are the most expressive area of the face, it is one of the first areas to wrinkle as you age. Moisturizing eye creams may not give you much more than a good, rich facial moisturizer would. Specialized eye creams, however, can deliver other benefits, like exfoliation, in a formula better suited to the eye area.

Select your eye cream according to your biggest concern. Get a tightening formula if you have puffiness, a moisturizing and exfoliating formula if the concern is wrinkles. The verdict is still out as to the effectiveness of undereye circle–diminishing creams (most of which, incidentally, contain an ingredient to help bruises heal faster!), but you can give it a try. Just don't expect miracles from this or any eye cream.

Eye creams are excellent for preparing the area for makeup application, as discussed in Chapter 4. They help to plump up lines and allow makeup to go on more smoothly. Since some eye cream formulations can be a little heavy, you might want to consider a lighter formula for daytime application.

Eating right

FOR YEARS PHYSICIANS HAVE MAINTAINED THAT HOW YOU EAT HAS NO EFFECT ON YOUR complexion. Telling teenagers to stay away from pizza and chocolate to minimize acne now seems old-fashioned. But the current interest in alternative health care and a holistic approach to health has had an impact on the beauty industry. There is no shortage of nutritionists and facialists to the stars who insist that a good diet with lots of water (at least eight 8 oz. glasses a day) are the key to keeping skin its clearest. Who to believe? The answer seems plain: Going easy on the *chicharrones* and ice cream sundaes and eating a healthy, well-balanced diet is essential for internal health and for feeling good about yourself. Respecting your body overall will make you feel good, and this will affect how you look. Period.

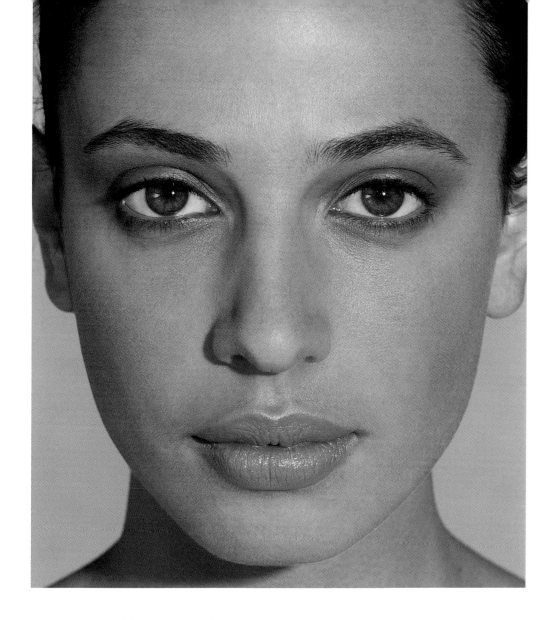

Extra Steps/Tips
For Every Skin Type

Dry

✔ Avoid soap-based cleansers, toners, astringents, and drying masks.

✔ Always use a moisturizer. Even dry skin can fall victim to acne, however, if the moisturizer is too oily.

✔ Do not use excessively hot water to wash or when you bathe. This exacerbates dryness.

Oily

✔ Toners, astringents, and other oil-cutting products may be useful to control overproduction of oil, which can lead to breakouts.

✔ Be careful to not overdry your skin, as this won't necessarily diminish

breakouts but will add arid, peeling skin to the mix, as well as subsequent over-production by the oil glands in areas like the T-zone.

✔ A relatively new topical product called Tazorac gel is available with a doctor's prescription. The gel shows promise in helping to control oil production.

✔ Use a moisturizer only when and where you need it. Make sure it is water-based, oil-free, and noncomedogenic.

✔ When you can, simply use a zinc oxide- or Parsol 1789–containing sunscreen and skip the moisturizer altogether.

Combination

✔ This is the trickiest skin to treat, since it is all about keeping things balanced. Fortunately, for most combo-skin types, the oiliness is centered in the T-zone area, where everyone has a higher concentration of sebaceous glands. Use a water-based, oil-free, noncomedogenic moisturizer, but only in the areas where you need it.

Acne solutions

AS MENTIONED IN THE "BEAUTY MYTH BUSTED!" on page 110, acne is caused by an excess of sebum, the waxy, oily substance produced by the oil glands that serves as the skin's natural moisturizer. As sebum travels from lower layers to the surface, it mixes with sticky skin cells and can get stuck and block the pores. The surrounding area may then become red and inflamed due to bacteria present in the skin. Hormonal fluctuations also contribute to acne breakouts by increasing sebum production.

One of the many aggravating things about acne is that spot treatments aren't always that effective. Treatments are meant to be applied to affected areas to prevent future outbreaks, but women often make the mistake of piling on a treatment over an existing pimple, excessively drying out the skin. Once a pimple is there, it has to run its course. The only option if you have a big one coming up on your face and an even bigger event (like a wedding or *quinceañera*) coming up in your life: Go to a dermatologist, who can inject the pimple with steroids that will make it go away temporarily. Even injected pimples, however, sometimes resurface.

In general, different types of acne respond better to different treatments. Here is a quick guide:

Blackheads: Contrary to popular belief, blackheads are not dirty pores; they are enlarged pores clogged with and darkened by sebum and sticky skin cells.

Blackheads are best treated with AHAs and BHAs to help slough off the top skin layer. Vitamin A–derived products may also help, since they get beneath the skin's surface and loosen blocked pores.

Whiteheads: These slightly raised blemishes are oils and dead skin cells trapped beneath the skin's surface in a pore and sealed over (which is why they do not appear dark). Like blackheads, whiteheads are best treated with AHAs and BHAs to help slough off the top skin layer; plus, they respond more dramatically to Vitamin A–derived products that loosen blocked pores.

Cysts: When whiteheads grow large, they become cysts, swellings beneath the skin's surface. Severe acne with many cysts below the skin's surface is referred to as cystic acne. Cystic acne should be treated by a dermatologist.

Papules: Red, inflamed bumps on the skin's surface. Benzoyl peroxide, an antibacterial that exfoliates the skin, unblocks pores, and dries up excess oil, is a good option. Prescription-only topical and oral antibiotics are also effective treatments for this type of acne.

Pustules: Pus-packed bumps on the skin's surface. These inflamed whiteheads surrounded by large red swelling are the most common type of acne formation. Benzoyl peroxide and prescription topical and oral antibiotics are the best treatments for this type of acne.

Sensitive

✔ Avoid products that feature extra ingredients like vitamin E, aloe vera, and, if you've determined them to be problematic (see "A Bad Acid Trip," p. 109) any type of acids (alpha hydroxy, beta hydroxy, and glycolic), which can aggravate sensitive skin.

✔ Stick to fragrance-free products.

Wrinkles

WRINKLES OCCUR FROM ACCUMULATED SUN DAMAGE AS WELL AS being a normal by-product of age. Aging causes the skin to lose some of its elasticity, which causes the sagging that appears as wrinkles, and gravity's pull on the muscles is also a factor. But sun exposure accelerates the aging process, which is why fairer-skinned Latinas, who are more prone to sun damage, tend to get more wrinkles than their darker-skinned *hermanas*.

The principal ways to combat the onset of "experience" lines:

✔ Regular use of a sunscreen with either Parsol 1789 or zinc or titanium oxide in the formula. (Staying out of the sun goes hand-in-hand with this.)

✔ Don't sleep on your face; those nightly hours of pressure do have a cumulative effect.

✔ Don't smoke. Smoke is one free radical you can eliminate (except in the form of secondhand smoke). If what cigarettes do to the inside of your body isn't enough, eschew them for wrinkle prevention.

Once you've got the wrinkle, options for minimizing its appearance are many:

✔ Prescriptions of Retin-A products applied nightly help to reduce fine wrinkles.

✔ Over-the-counter items with retinol contain Retin-A in less potent amounts, but can still be beneficial.

✔ AHAs also help to reduce fine lines by increasing exfoliation and stimulating collagen and elastin growth in the deeper layers.

✔ Products with anti-oxidants give preventive care due to their free radical–fighting powers.

Facials

SOME *MUJERES* SWEAR BY THEIR MONTHLY FACIALS, ALTHOUGH most dermatologists traditionally maintain that facials have no real long-term impact on improving the skin or on fighting wrinkles. Things are slowly evolving, however, as more and more dermatologists are beginning to offer the services of specially trained estheticians to their clients. Whether you get your facial through a doctor's office or through a spa or salon, some general guidelines apply.

What a good facial will definitely do: leave you feeling pampered, well moisturized, and deep-cleaned. Select a facialist with the same caution you would a manicurist. They must use clean utensils (towels, latex gloves, etc.) for each new customer, especially in terms of utensils used for extractions.

One word on extractions: When a facialist is extracting blackheads, or squeezing out trapped impurities from clogged pores, slight discomfort is normal. Pain, however, is not. Pimple popping or blackhead removal that is so overzealous it hurts can lead to scarring.

Deep-cleansing facial

What it is: A gentle cleansing massage that unclogs pores and exfoliates the dead skin cells on the surface, leaving the skin thoroughly cleansed and moisturized.

Procedure: Skin is cleansed, then massaged. Next, a steam machine may be directed toward the face for a few minutes to open pores. Clogged pores (blackheads and whiteheads) are then extracted. Finally, facial mask is smoothed and left on the skin for a few minutes to tighten pores again, then washed off and followed by a moisturizer.

Good for: All skin types except oily.

Glycolic facial

What it is: This facial expands on the deep-cleansing facial with the addition of glycolic acid, which enhances exfoliation and improves skin tone and texture.

Procedure: Same as deep-cleansing facial, except glycolic acid is applied after extraction.

Good for: Most skin types, especially those with sun damage, but not recommended for those with highly sensitive skin.

Oily skin facial

What it is: An adaptation of the deep-cleansing facial, an oily skin facial involves less facial massage, which can stimulate oil glands.

Procedure: Similar to the deep-cleansing facial, except that oily skin facials use only oil-free products and include the use of astringents.

Good for: Oily, combination, or acne-prone skin.

Manchas and Skin-Lightening Creams

MANCHAS, HYPERPIGMENTATION OF THE SKIN, CAN BE GENETIC OR can develop as a result of hormonal influences or skin inflammation. They are further aggravated by exposure to the sun.

Manchas caused by hormones can be brought on by pregnancy (called melasma, or the mask of pregnancy) or from taking birth-control pills. These types of *manchas* tends to be blotchier and larger than the sun spots and freckles caused by sun exposure, another cause of these discolorations. Sun exposure *manchas* generally appear on women in their 30s and are

Refreshing bath treatment:
Add ¼ cup apple cider vinegar plus 5 drops of your favorite essential oil to warm bathwater. After a 15- to 20-minute bath, apply a body oil to damp skin. Skin will feel toned and pampered.

accentuated and made more apparent after any length of time spent in the sun without sunscreen. The third cause of *manchas* is post-inflammatory hyperpigmentation, when dark brown marks remain on the skin after inflammations such as a bug bite or a pimple. The deposit of the pigment is deeper in these cases and can take a longer time to fade whether treated or untreated.

Manchas do fade with time, but you can speed the process with a regular, strict regimen of skin-lightening cream and sunblock. A good skin-lightening cream (also called fade cream) can be purchased over the counter. Stronger fade creams can be obtained with a prescription.

One common myth about *manchas* is that they only appear on women with darker skin tones. This untruth can have disastrous effects for fair-skinned Latinas who have laser treatments or chemical peels done by doctors or estheticians unfamiliar with how to avoid post-inflammatory hyperpigmentation. While on fair-skinned Latinas, *manchas* may start out red before turning brown, make no mistake about it—it's a *mancha*, and it may or may not go away even with a good skin-lightening cream.

Skin lightening creams are to be used only on dark hyperpigmented spots. Made with 2 percent hydroquinone, a topical agent that inhibits melanin production, they are certainly not meant to be used all over the face or as an attempt to change the color of one's skin.

Because of our tendency to develop hyperpigmentation, especially post-inflammatory hyperpigmentation, we must carefully consider cosmetic treatments Caucasian women undergo without a second thought. Procedures such as electrolysis, laser skin resurfacing, and even laser hair removal should be done with the utmost caution.

What tells you it's time to go to a dermatologist?

• The sudden appearance of, or change in, a skin growth or sore, especially if it bleeds easily or does not seem to heal.

• A rash that has lasted longer than a week and persists despite repeated application of an over-the-counter topical cream meant to cure or minimize it.

• Acne that has not responded to a consistently applied over-the-counter topical treatment after four weeks.

• Sensitive skin types that develop rashes in response to necessary skin-care elements (i.e., cleanser,

moisturizer, sun protection) that do not contain perfume, are noncomedogenic, and are described as "safe for sensitive skin."

• Either very early (12 or 13) or late (early 20s) development of acne. Early development of acne may predict more severe acne at a later date which can be prevented or controlled with early intervention. Adult acne is usually caused by hormonal changes and should also be taken care of under a doctor's supervision, as adult-onset acne tends to be resistant to over-the-counter treatments.

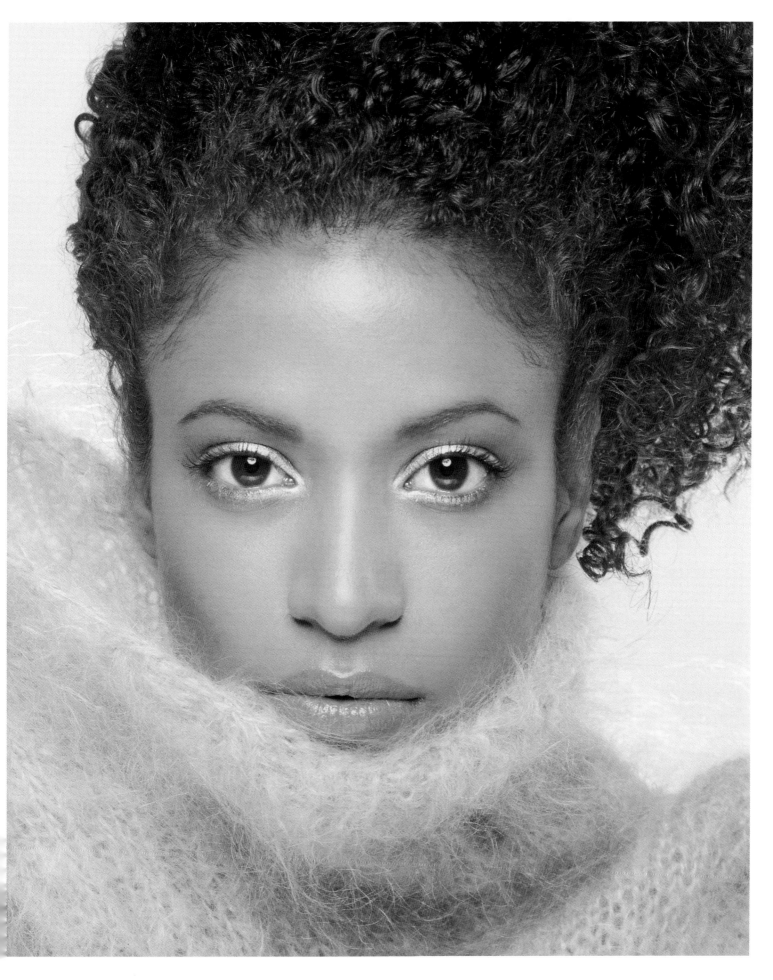

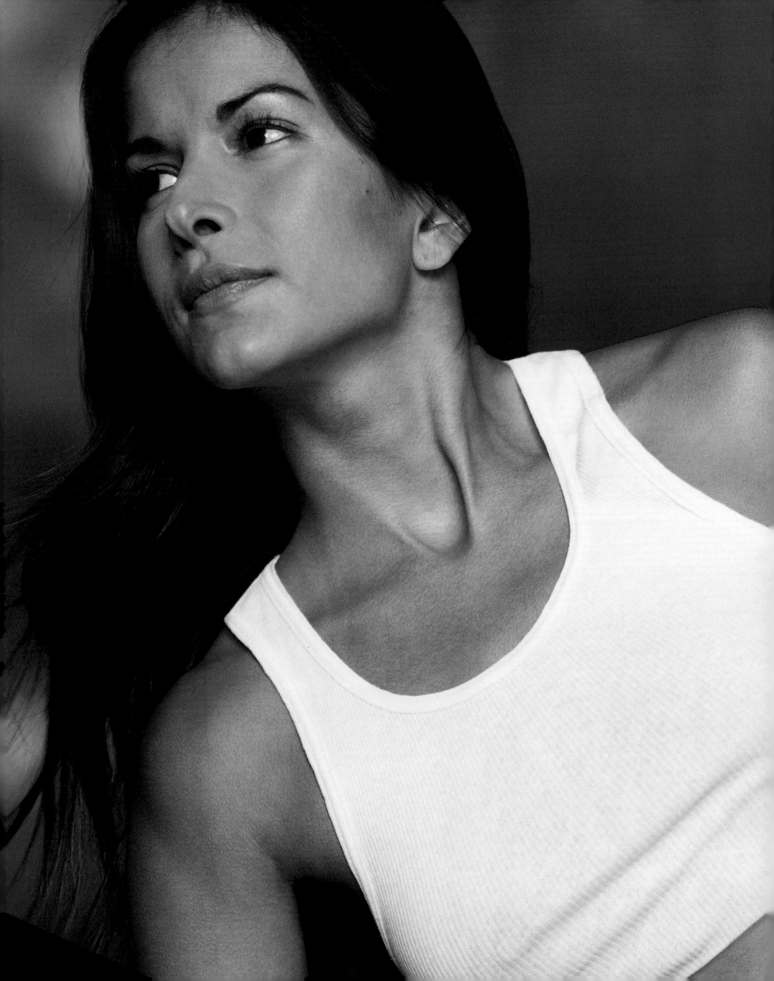

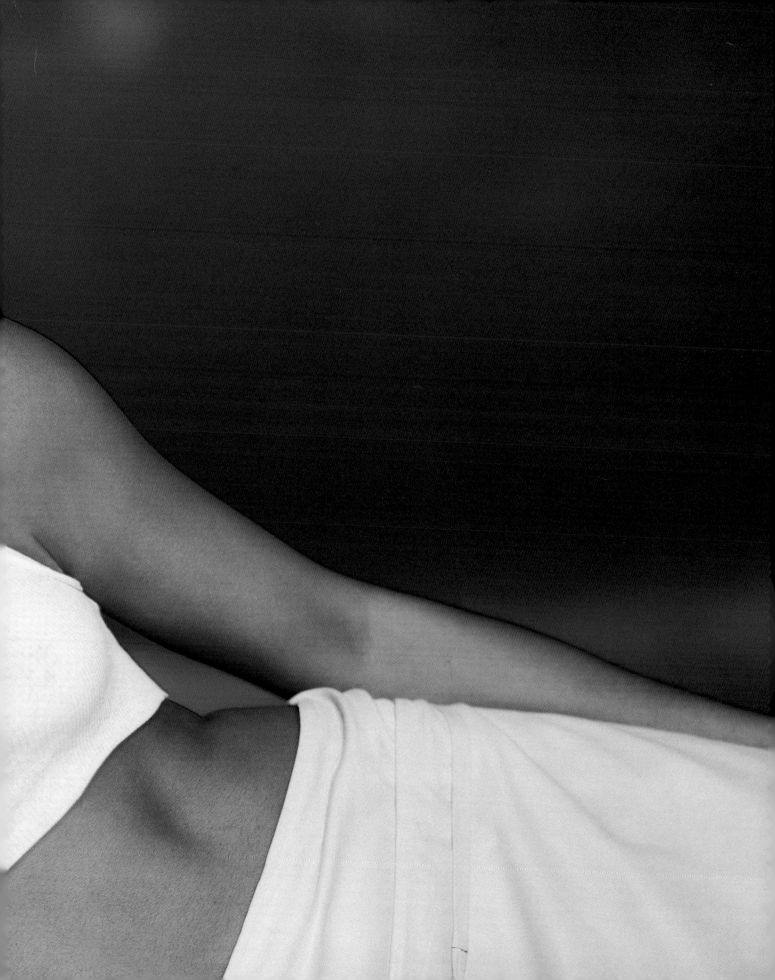

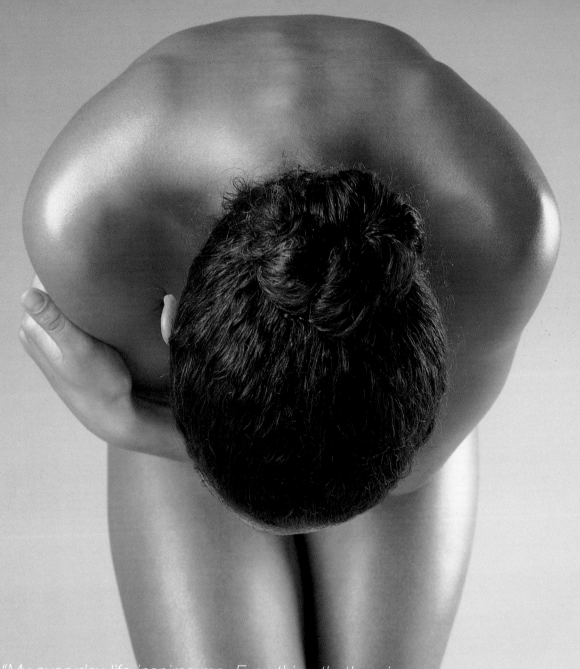

"My everyday life inspires me. Everything that's going on around you inspires—your children, the way you live, going to museums, reading a book, listening to music, seeing people. Being alive is an inspiration."
—CAROLINA HERRERA

Skin Care
From the Neck Down

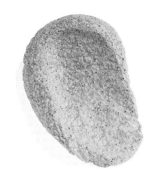

Cleansing

Use a regular, gentle soap for parts of the body that don't need extra moisturizing—the underarms, the feet, and, if you have problems with acne, the back and chest. Antibacterial soaps can also be used in these areas for short periods of time (like during the summer) if you want extra protection. Excessive usage, however, can cause irritation or overgrowth of the wrong types of bacteria on the skin.

Body washes or a moisturizing bar soap are the best choices for the rest of the body. Select them according to your heart's desires. Indulge in fragrances you like.

Just like facial skin, skin on the body shows signs of stress and aging. Proper care keeps it glowing and pampered-looking.

Exfoliating

As mentioned before, body creams with AHAs do the work of exfoliation for you, but why use them exclusively when exfoliating with a scrub, loofah, or body brush can feel so good? Body exfoliation is only needed three times a week at the most. Scrubs now come in so many different fragrances and formulations you can experiment until you find what you like. The only rule for exfoliation is that it should feel great on the skin; if you feel like you're being scrubbed with wet cement or your skin feels irritated, stop. The benefits of exfoliation below the neck? Your body feels smooth, fresh, and sexy afterward.

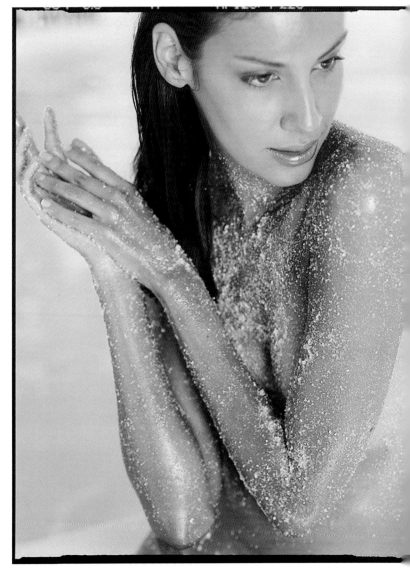

Moisturizing

Unlike the face, where moisturizing is optional depending on skin type, almost everyone needs a little cream on their legs pretty regularly. Besides, moisturizing, like cleansing, should be a moment, however brief, of pure indulgence and pampering. Yield to whims, curiosity, and experimentation when it comes to body creams. As long as it gets the job done—keeping your skin smooth, supple, and well-hydrated, why not try different formulas? Those with sensitive skin, however, need to be more cautious.

You may find that your legs and arms need different moisturizers for different times of the year. A heavier cream or oil keeps ashiness away during winter, while a lighter lotion is good for summer.

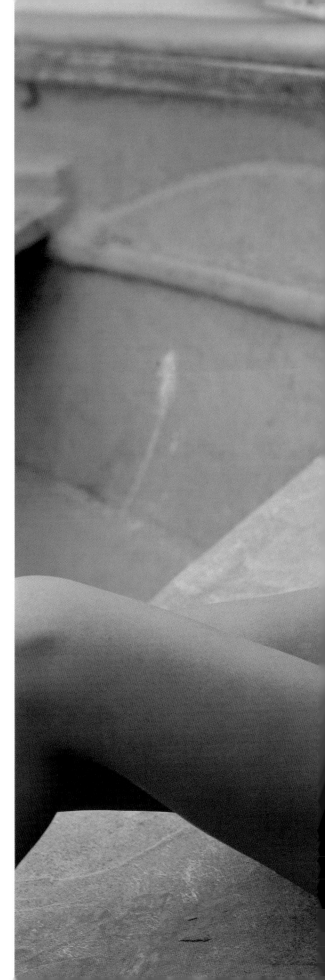

SPF

The rest of your body, like your face, does need regular sun protection as well. As a rule, SPF formulas should be applied to any area exposed to the sun.

The hands, which like the face are exposed virtually year-round, are particularly susceptible to sun damage. Because of this, you may want to consider investing in a special hand cream that protects as a regular sunscreen would but also has added benefits. In addition to moisturizing the skin, more hand creams are also incorporating AHAs into the formula, helping to diminish sunspots and other signs of aging.

Stretch marks

Stretch marks can appear after rapid weight loss or gain. They occur when the elastic tissue within the skin's deeper layers gets broken. While there is no cure for stretch marks once they appear, they can be minimized with lasers or with Retin-A. Even these techniques, however, are only effective on red stretch marks, and even then they will only diminish their appearance, not erase them. If you are pregnant or undergoing a rapid weight loss or weight gain or are in an early-teens growth spurt, keep the skin well moisturized. Remember to apply the cream to breasts as well.

Varicose veins

Varicose veins are a largely inherited trait that can be exacerbated by certain lifestyle factors, such as being overweight, standing for long numbers of hours during the day, or sitting for hours with your legs crossed. The best treatment for varicose veins is sclerotherapy, which involves having a concentrated solution injected directly into the vein, causing the vein to collapse. Support hose are then worn for a prescribed amount of time afterward. Scelerotherapy works best on small veins. For large, knotted, and painful varicose veins, the only option may be venous stripping or actual removal of the veins— a more expensive and difficult procedure.

As with stretch marks, the best defense is prevention: a healthy, active lifestyle in which long periods of standing, sitting crosslegged, and prolonged weight gain are avoided. The vitamin supplement horse chestnut extract is believed to be effective at preventing the further development of varicose veins. Once there, however, the only way to remove them is to undergo surgery or injections.

Laser treatments, a relatively new technique to minimize small varicose veins or spider veins, are preferable for fair-skinned Latinas, since the laser treatments may cause pigment changes in darker skin types. Again, as with any laser work, care should be taken to ensure that the practitioner has experience working with women of color.

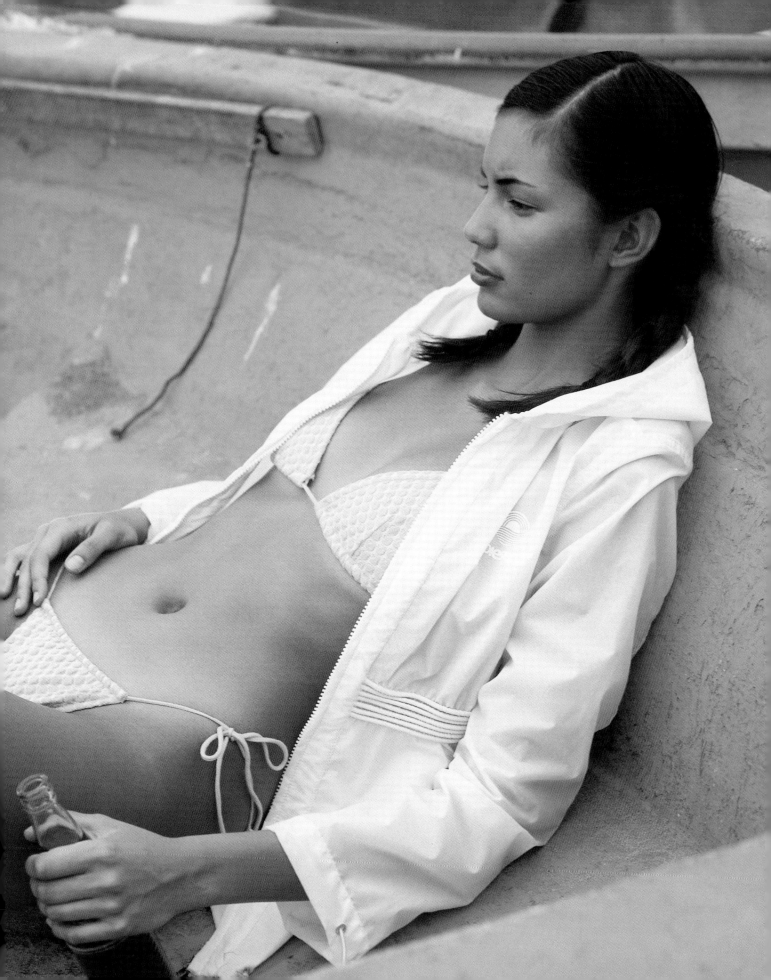

Facial Hair Removal

HAIR REMOVAL ON THE FACE REQUIRES A DIFFERENT APPROACH THAN removal of body hair. Also, for some Latinas, facial-hair removal isn't isolated to the standard eyebrow and *bigote* removal, since many also elect to remove the baby hairs along the hairline and cheeks.

For short-term removal, consider the following.

• If your facial hair is particularly noticeable or thick, try going to a medical doctor to make sure there is no hormonal imbalance at work, which could lead to far more severe medical consequences. Hormonal treatments are available that diminish hair thickness.

• Shaving, especially of facial hairs that are thick and/or wiry, is not recommended as a method of removal. Regrowth could cause ingrown hairs, which can lead to acne-like bumps on the skin, scarring, and hyperpigmentation.

• Waxing is the best option for removing facial hair, since the hairs are grabbed from the root and regrowth takes longer (four to five weeks). The hair also regrows softly, without the thick stubble shaving produces.

As mentioned in Chapter 4 (page 57), women who do facial waxing and are also using strong Retin-A-based acne medicine should stop applying the cream three to four days before getting waxed. Retin-A sloughs off the skin's excess outer layers, leaving it susceptible to rawness and irritation.

Again, if you break out after getting waxed, especially along the cheeks, hairline, and upper lip, do not allow the esthetician to apply a heavy cream over the area after the hair has been removed. Follow with an astringent to make sure the skin is not infected, and simply let the skin air-dry or follow with an application of aloe vera gel to soothe the area.

Threading

This method of hair removal, that involves moving tightly coiled thread quickly across the face to remove the hairs from the root, is another good option. It eliminates the heat factor of hot wax, so skin is not so sensitive and irritated afterward. Threading is not as widely available as waxing, so check out local hair salons to see who offers the procedure.

Bleaching

This is an option if the hairs themselves are not too thick, coarse, or long, and if your complexion is not too dark. The browner you are, the more likely that you will simply give yourself an orange moustache instead of eliminating your black one. For honey-skinned girls, you may be able to get away with leaving the bleaching mixture on for less time, but it's a tricky method. If you overbleach, the whole world can see it. It's probably better to stick to waxing or threading.

For long-term hair removal or permanent hair reduction, two options exist:

Electrolysis

Electrolysis involves having the tip of a needle inserted into the tiny hair follicle. An electric current is then sent through the needle into the skin, destroying the

---

Mami **says:** "Cocoa butter prevents stretch marks."

Doctor says: True, some of the time. According to Victor Beraja, M.D., a Miami-based plastic surgeon, stretch marks can be prevented depending on your type of skin. "Stretch marks are caused by a break in collagen fibers and blood vessels, usually spurred by fast weight gain or rapid growth," he notes. "The thicker, darker, and more elastic your skin, the more resistant it is."

Oily, thick, and creamy moisturizers, like baby oil or cocoa butter, can increase the elasticity of your skin, Dr. Beraja says, adding that massaging also stimulates circulation, which prevents a break in blood vessels.

Beauty myth **busted!**

Hair removal

Shaving

Description: A razor is used to cut hair at the surface of the skin.

Best for: Women with thin, fine, or light-colored body hair. The legs and underarms respond best to this method.

Cost: $2–$5 for a high-quality razor. Invest in a good, rich shaving cream that will help to avoid nicks or cuts.

Duration: Two to three days

Be careful of:

• Nicks, cuts, and dull blades. Clean the blade by tapping it against a clean surface to loosen tiny hairs. Never clean razors with a washcloth; this dulls the blade and could lead to nicks.

• Ingrown hairs in the bikini area; use a lotion that specifically prevents in-growns after shaving.

• Shaving while using a self-tanner. Since shaving exfoliates the top layer of skin, where tanner leaves its pigment, you could end up with stripes along your legs.

Depilatory

Description: A cream-based chemical preparation that disintegrates hair.

Best for: Women with medium to light amounts of body hair. Most successful on legs and arms.

Cost: $5–$7 per bottle.

Duration: Up to a week.

Be careful of:

• Leaving the depilatory on the skin too long, which can burn the top layer. Be especially careful when doing areas like the bikini line, where hair is coarser and the tendency is to leave the solution on longer. Test on a small area first.

Waxing

Description: There are different types of waxes, but the most commonly used in this country is honey-based. The wax must be warmed and applied in thin layers to the skin in the same direction of the hair growth. A strip of muslin or cotton cloth is placed over the waxed area and removed the with one brisk tug in the opposite direction of hair growth, bringing with it hairs pulled from the root.

Best for: Women with dark, thicker body hair or fair-skinned women on whom hair regrowth caused by shaving is quickly noticeable. The legs, arms, face, toes, fingers are the best areas for this method.

Cost: Home kits can cost around $10. For the first time, it's better to go to a salon, where a full leg and bikini wax can run up to $80.

Duration: Three to four weeks, depending on how quickly your hair grows. Hair grows at different rates on different parts of the body. The bikini line grows the fastest, with some women having to book appointments every two weeks. The areas of the legs below the knee also tend to grow faster.

Be careful of:

• Applying lotion to skin the same day you will be waxed. Skin should be as dry as possible—some estheticians sprinkle a layer of baby powder on the legs before waxing so that the wax grips the hair firmly.

• Getting waxed at the wrong time in your cycle. Right before menstruation the skin can become particularly sensitive, and waxing at this time is excruciating for some women.

• Ingrown hair regrowth. Buy a special lotion for the bikini area. Regular exfoliation with a loofah or body scrub should be enough for the rest of the body. Wait a week before exfoliating after you wax.

Sugaring

Description: Not as widely available as waxing, this method involves having a mixture of sugar applied to the skin. The mixture is pliable, like Silly Putty. It is rolled over the skin, almost like a ball, removing hair from the root as it goes over the surface of the skin. It is said to be less painful than waxing

Best for: Women with dark, thicker body hair and fair-skinned women, for whom regrowth from shaving is a more immediate problem. The legs, arms, and face are the best areas for this method.

Cost: $10–$80, depending on how much you are having done.

Duration: Same as with waxing

Be careful of:

• Ingrown hairs during regrowth, as with waxing, since both procedures remove hair from the root.

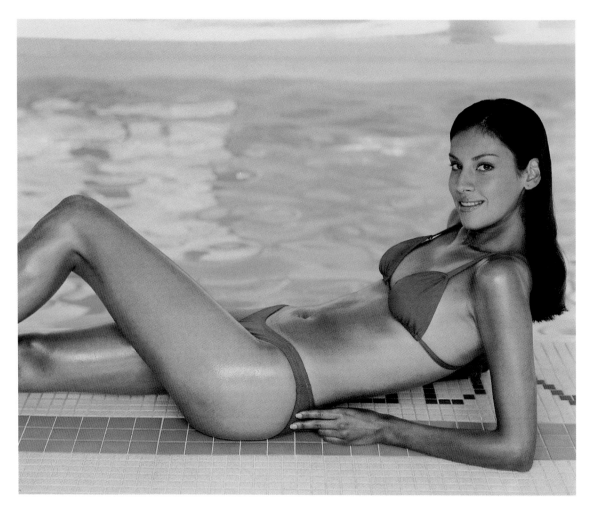

Bikini basics

WHEN IT COMES TO THE DELICATE BIKINI AREA, the best method of hair removal depends on the amount of hair you have to remove and on the sensitivity of the skin.

Generally, waxing provides the longest hair-free period of all the temporary methods.

• Don't take aspirin as a painkiller before the waxing session. Aspirin thins the blood and can lead to increased bleeding or bruising. Take ibuprofen instead.

• If your pubic hairs are particularly long, trim them down to a manageable length before getting waxed. You want the esthetician to get a clean shape, and at all costs you want to avoid having to remove any extra hair unnecessarily. If the area is trimmed and tidy, it makes the waxer's job that much easier.

• Use your bikini or underwear bottoms as a guide for the type of wax you should get. If you wear bottoms with a generous cut, there is no need to get a bikini wax that goes particularly deep. If you decide to be *brava* and wear a thong poolside, commit to a Brazilian style bikini wax. Brazilian bikini waxes leave you completely bare except for a landing-strip-type piece in front. Expect to go to the waxing salon, take off your underwear, and have your legs spread into all kinds of strange positions. This method is not for *muchachas* with a low threshold for pain.

• Ingrown hairs in the bikini area may be persistent and unresponsive to loofah or regular exfoliation. If this is the case, buy a topical lotion or an astringent formulated to prevent ingrown hairs. If ingrowns leave you with post-inflammatory hyperpigmentation, a twice-daily application of skin-lightening cream on the affected spots fade them.

hair bulb under the skin where the hair grows. The process is painful and can result in scabbing at the hair follicle.

The knowledge that scabbing is involved raises a red flag for women of color. Many Latinas respond to scabbing by developing hyperpigmentation, brown spots that draw attention to the scab. Arm yourself with a generous supply of skin-lightening cream. Start applying the lightening cream at least one month before the procedure as a preventative step. Also, for Latinas who have problems with keloids (raised, bumpy scarring), a trip to the electrolysist can leave a nasty trace.

If you are really committed to having electrolysis done anyway, go to an electrolysist who has a lot of experience doing the procedure on people of color. You may also want to try it on less visible parts of the body (such as the bikini line) to see how the skin there responds, before having the procedure done on the face.

Laser hair removal

Approved by the FDA as a method of "permanent hair reduction," this expensive (and considerably less painful than electrolysis) procedure merits a few words of caution.

• The FDA defined "permanent" hair reduction as lasting at least one and a half to two years—in other words, not a lifetime. Be aware that laser hair removal requires a minimum of three visits throughout the first year and a few follow-up visits that could be ongoing (though sporadic) thereafter.

• Laser hair removal works best for women who are fair-skinned with very dark hair, since, to put it very simply, the lasers do their work through detecting the differences in pigment between the skin and the hair. Hence, the greater the difference, the more effective this option will be. For light-skinned, dark haired women, a long-pulse ruby laser may be the best option. Darker-skinned Latinas should avoid this laser, as it can cause a loss of pigmentation (hypopigmentation) on darker skin tones.

• Diode lasers that emit wavelengths in the very high 800 range are used on darker-skinned patients. The diode laser is highly effective, achieving about an 80 percent reduction in hair growth.

• The bottom line on lasers: This is rapidly developing technology. It may be a better idea to wait and see what developments take place in using lasers for hair removal. Since skin discoloration is a concern with laser hair removal, stick with an expert who has experience on his or her side. Newer methods of permanent hair removal or creams which can be used in conjunction with lasers may be approved by the FDA as soon as winter 2000. It may be a good idea to simply wait until the technology develops further.

If you do decide to experiment with lasers, go to a dermatologist or plastic surgeon instead of an esthetician. Also, make sure that the doctor has experience specifically treating women of color with lasers.

Mami **says:** "If you shave your body hair, it will grow back stronger and thicker."

Doctor says: Absolutely not true. According to Mary Ann Martinez, M.D., a dermatologist in Austin, Texas, when stubble grows back, its initial roughness makes it seem thicker. "When you shave, you are just cutting the hair," Dr. Martinez says. "It comes back with the same density it had originally."

Beauty myth **busted!**

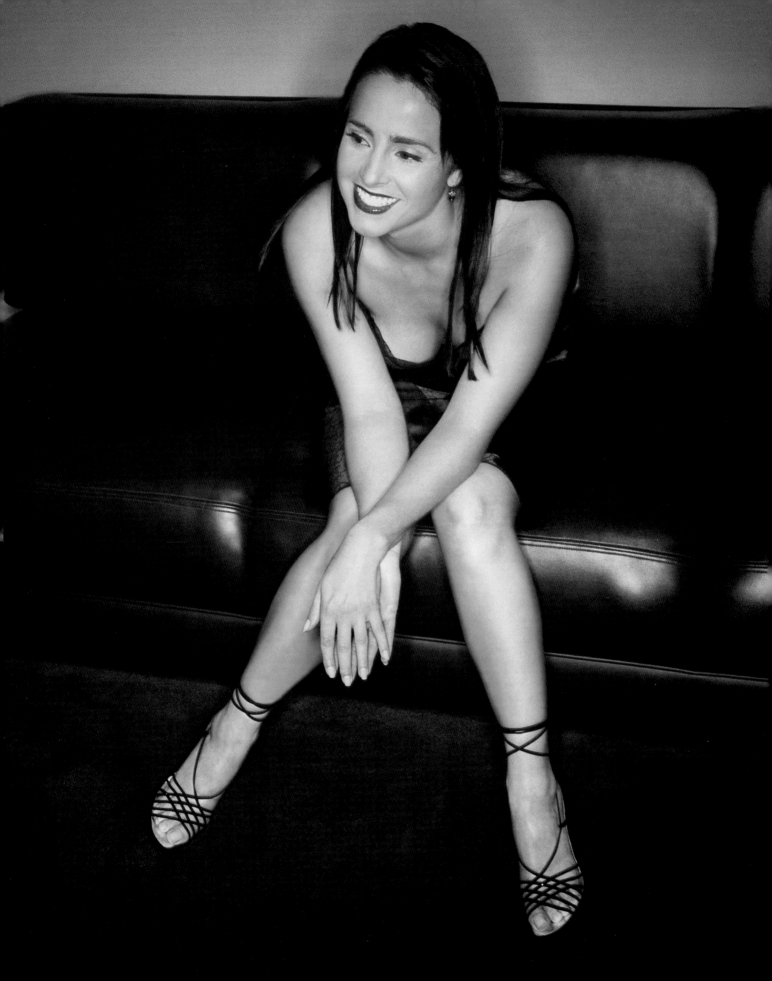

Hand to Toe

YOU DON'T HAVE TO BE A *BRUJA* TO KNOW A LOT ABOUT A WOMAN FROM HOW SHE KEEPS her fingernails. Forget palm reading; nail reading tells people whether you take the time to take care of yourself or spend too much time—and money—on the artificial. (Women with nail carvings or those charms hanging from the nail tips, for example, would fall into the latter group.)

The feet are revealing as well. We all know women who keep their *uñas* workmanlike, plain and short, only to reveal a pair of well-kept feet with sexy siren-red toenails. If your feet look as neglected and taken for granted as your comfy, raggedy house *chanclas*, make the time to turn your hands and feet into the sexy, smooth appendages they were meant to be.

En La Casa Nail Care

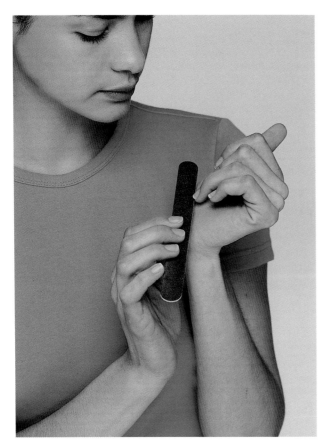

Manicures are easy to do at home and provide a way to pamper yourself. Two important tools (below): A fine-grain nail file and cuticle cream.

1) Remove polish.

Believe it or not, there is a proper way to do it. This method may appear to take more time but in the end actually saves trouble, since you won't have to swipe up the excess polish that the remover can leave caked in the cuticles and hard-to-reach spaces on the nail surface.

✔ Saturate the cotton ball with remover. You should have enough in it so that when you apply the cotton ball to the nail, the soaked area covers the entire face and edges of the nail.

✔ Place the saturated cotton ball on the nail, applying very slight pressure.

✔ Leave the cotton ball on the entire nail and nail bed for a count of about 30 seconds.

✔ Lift off the cotton ball. The polish should come almost entirely off with the cotton. If you have applied two layers of top coat plus additional layers throughout the week to keep the manicure fresh, you may have to repeat the procedure.

2) Shape the nail.

After the polish is off, you are ready to shape the nails. You probably already know that if you file each nail in one direction only toward the center of the nail, you will prevent your nails from splitting and peeling. Most *mujeres* simply choose to saw back and forth on their poor nails anyway. We can't blame you; it's quicker and easier to shape the nail this way. In truth, the most common mistake you can make when shaping the nails isn't only the back-and-forth motion of the file, it's also the type of file you use. Throw out and ban from your house those old-fashioned metal files. Instead, invest in a good-quality fine-grain emery board. Files are basically sandpaper. Just as you use a fine-grain sandpaper to give a nice finish to wood, a fine-grain nail file will shape your nails smoothly, causing minimal splitting or peeling.

The only rules for shaping are personal taste and the health of your nails. Women should decide for themselves whether they prefer a classic, oval shape or the more modern, short, square shape. You are also the best judge of the appropriate length for your nails. In any case, avoid filing the sides and corners of the nail. Doing so could result in an ingrown nail. Also, as the nail grows longer, the sides tend to curve in anyway. By filing down the corner you weaken the nail, making it more prone to breakage.

3) Apply cuticle cream.

In most salons, nail polish removal is followed by a quick soak of the fingertips in warm water to soften the cuticles. Since few of us have the time or patience for this step when we do a manicure at home, a thick, emollient hand or cuticle cream is a good substitute. Simply apply the cream to the cuticle area, massaging it gently into the nail bed and over the nail itself.

4) Push back the cuticles.

There is no reason, if you take regular care of your nails, that you should ever have to cut your cuticles. The cuticles serve a purpose: They protect the nail root. Regularly, gently pushing them back eliminates the need to cut cuticles and all the problems cuticle-cutting can present. The best instruments for keeping cuticles under control is a wooden stick, a rubber-topped pusher, or a pumice cuticle pusher. Along with the aforementioned metal nail file, throw out those old metal cuticle pushers. They are far too harsh and are often ineffective. If you go to a salon that attempts to push back your cuticles with a metal pusher, insist they use the gentle pumice version or the wooden stick.

5) Trim any hangnails.

Cuticle clippers are useful, however, when it comes to hangnails—that's why you should get one. If not cut quickly and at the source, hangnails can get bigger and worse, so keep the cuticle cutter handy. A high-quality cuticle cutter will cut the hangnail cleanly and evenly, with no additional tugging or pulling.

6) Use the nail polish remover again.

Most manicurists follow trimming the hangnails with a second quick wipe of nail polish remover. This is because the nail itself needs to be dry in order to hold the enamels you will be putting on it, and because polish remover also takes out any residual oils from the cuticle or hand cream.

7) Apply a base coat.

When giving yourself a home manicure, it is well worth the trouble to apply a base coat to the nail, especially if you are using a dark color that will easily be noticeable if chipped. A base coat, like a top coat,

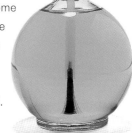

More manicure must-have's (top to bottom): Pumice cuticle pusher, wood cuticle sticks, and base coat.

Lujoso vs. *bueno, bonito, y barato*

WHEN IT COMES TO THE HANDS, "SPLURGING" involves going to a beauty supply store to purchase a few professional-quality implements. The tools will last a lifetime, but they won't break the bank. The rest of the items can be purchased at any drugstore.

Splurge:
- high-quality cuticle clipper
- nonacetone nail polish remover
- fine-grain nail file
- pumice cuticle pusher (or wooden stick, see below)

Save:
- wooden stick
- base coat
- color
- top coat
- quick-dry oil
- cotton balls

is one of the first steps women doing at-home home manicures skip in an effort to save time This can actually cost you time later in the week. Most base coats do basic things like strengthen the nail itself by offering more protection. But they also help to prepare the nail for color, providing a smooth surface color adheres to longer. A base coat also helps prevent discoloration or yellowing of the nail, a cause for concern to women who often wear dark colors on their nails.

8) Apply color.

With the wide variety of colors on the market today, from bright green to the always-sexy classic red, options abound. One tip to make polish last longer: Mix a few drops of nail polish remover into the nail polish if the consistency gets too thick and is hard to apply. Thickened, old nail polish also takes longer to dry.

There is a "right" way to apply color, too: Make sure you have the correct amount of polish on the brush to begin with. Newer polishes tend to be more fluid, so as you remove the brush from the bottle, gently smooth some of the excess polish off at the bottle's lip. Then, to avoid ending up with a thick, gooey, half-dried coat of old polish on the neck of the bottle, slightly lift the brush away as you come to its tip. This also helps polish last longer, as it allows you to keep a tight seal on the bottle when you close it.

Start at the nail base and apply one firm stroke of color down the middle of the nail. Then do the sides, which should be done with one stroke each. If you make a mistake, quickly take the pointed edge of the wooden stick and run it along the side of the nail to clean up excess polish. Some people wait until they have finished all the nails to clean up mistakes, but polish cleans up quite easily if you do it immediately after coloring each nail. After applying the first coat to all ten nails, follow with the second.

9) Use a top coat.

A base coat plus color is a manicure half-done. A top coat is what really makes the manicure last, but it is important to use both base and top coat together to get the most effective results.

One note about quick-dry oils, sprays, and even top coats: A lot of *hermanas* in a hurry apply the quick-dry coat, wait the recommended one minute, then proceed to carry on with whatever it is they have to do. A quick-dry coat dries the top layers of the nails, allowing you to resume most of your regular activity. Anything that actually applies pressure to the surface of the nail—buttoning up a pair of too-tight jeans, putting on a pair of gloves, banging your nails accidentally against a hard or pointed surface—will cause a *mancha* on the surface of the nails. No matter how quickly or effectively your quick-dry coat works, it still takes time for the layers of enamel to harden, as you may know if you've ever given yourself a manicure at night and woken up in the morning with sheet marks across your nails. Allow at least one hour for nail enamels to harden fully.

Bubble trouble

GETTING TINY BUBBLES ON YOUR POLISH AS it dries on your nails? It could be you shake it too much. A good nail polish doesn't need to be shaken vigorously. Simply roll the bottle between the palms of your hands two to three times. If the color doesn't seem to blend effectively after that—especially if it is a formula with shimmer in it—the polish may be too old. Add a few drops of nail polish remover to thin the formula and roll the bottle again. If this does not help, the polish is either no longer good or not good quality and should be thrown away.

A good top coat applied every two days will ensure that your manicure lasts for a week.

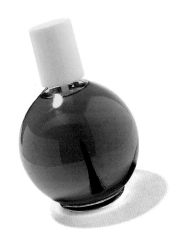

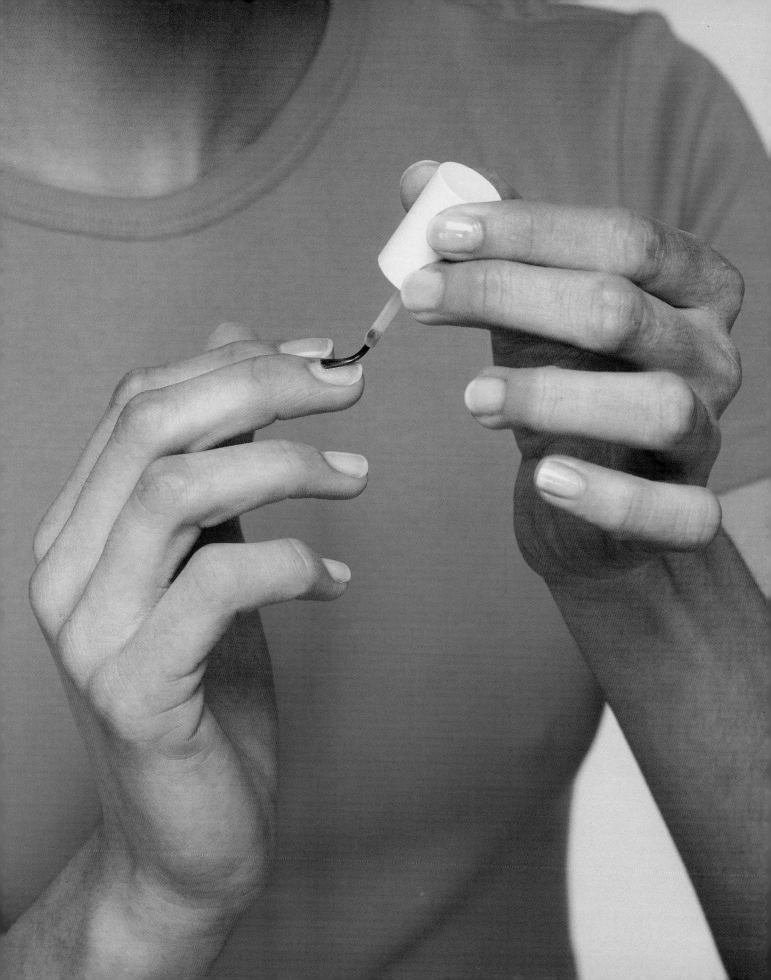

Fake Fingernails

THERE ARE MANY TECHNIQUES FOR ACHIEVING A PERFECT SET OF *uñas*, each with its own set of advantages and disadvantages. Below, the most common ways to purchase—and keep—beautiful nails.

Wraps

Wraps build upon the natural nail to improve strength and encourage growth without breakage. The benefit of getting nail wraps as opposed to acrylic tips is that wraps can also be used to mend a nail that is chipped or split but still mostly intact. Wraps can be used in conjunction with tips to extend the length of the natural nail, and some women think wraps look more "natural." This is a topic of some debate, however, as other nail estheticians maintain that acrylics, in fact, are less artificial-looking.

The natural nail is prepared much as at the beginning of a manicure (polish removed and cuticles pushed back), then the surface is roughened slightly with a file. Adhesive material, most commonly liquid nail glue, is applied to the nail with a brush. Next, wrapping material is cut to fit and placed over the entire nail, or over the chipped area, if the wrap is being used to repair a broken nail. (Some wrapping materials come precut and backed with adhesive, eliminating the need for the first round of glue.) Nail glue is then applied to adhere the material to the natural nail, creating a tight seal. The material is trimmed again and smoothed down to form a bond between the natural nail and the wrap itself. Wraps last about two weeks.

If you are adding fake extensions to the nail, tips are glued on the ends of the natural nail before the wrapping material. The material wraps over the natural nail and the tip. Glue and nail powder are then generously applied over the wrap to create a smooth surface. To level it further, you must have the surface of the nail very well filed.

Acrylic tips

Acrylic tips are becoming increasingly popular. Jennifer Lopez keeps hers in a French manicure style. Most women like them because they keep a manicure for as long as two weeks. Like wraps, however, they require regular upkeep. With acrylic tips, a plastic nail extension is fitted to the natural nail, adhered, and then smoothed over with an acrylic overlay or a bonding powder that forms into a paste when mixed with acetone.

The nail is prepared in a similar way as for wraps: Polish is removed, the cuticle area is pushed back, and the surface of the nail is filed down. Nail primer is then applied, an important step because primers contain ingredients that sterilize the nail area in order to prevent fungal infection. After primer has been

Beauty myth busted!

***Mami* says:** "Eat lots of gelatin to make your nails grow stronger."
Nutritionist says: Nails need protein, which gelatin has. But then again, so do many foods. "You can get it from other food sources, like meat, dairy, and vegetables," says Martha M. Dominguez, a nutritionist at the Women's Health Center in San Francisco. "Sometimes you'll find gelatin in nail polish, but all it really does is act as a protective coating for the nail. A polish without gelatin would serve the same function."

Did you **know?** Latinas are three times more likely than non-Hispanic women to use fake fingernails.

applied, the only thing that should touch the nail surface is the brush that contains the acrylic. Make sure your nail technician is careful and very clean.

After the nail is fitted and glued, the seam where the fake and natural nails meet is buffed with a file. Acrylic is then used to form a smooth bond between the natural nail and the tip. When the acrylic is dry and the surface of the bonded nail buffed smooth, polish is applied.

Acrylic nails must be maintained with regular visits to the manicurist every two weeks.

Fake nails for first-timers

If you are getting fake nails for the first time, you may be surprised at a few things. First, the chemicals used to perform either nail technique described above are abrasive and strong-smelling, as anyone who has ever walked into a salon specializing in artificial nails can tell you. Seeing a nail technician file down your natural nail can also be startling, since it seems to defy everything we have been taught about what to do to keep nails strong.

The condition of nails after tips have been removed can also be an unsettling sight. In some cases, the natural nail is weakened and soft, while in other cases the difference between new nail regrowth and the area where the acrylic overlay had been is clearly visible and, to say the least, unattractive. This happens when the nail technician has filed the natural nail too much prior to applying the adhesive or acrylic overlay. A good technician will file just enough to allow the adhesive to take hold. Unavoidably, the part of the nail that has been filed will look different from the part that hasn't, but not so much that a standard manicure won't cover it all smoothly. If the difference is so dramatic that a manicure won't cover it, that means the manicurist who did the original application of false nails filed excessively and you should not seek out her services again.

The worst-case scenario is fungal infection, which can happen even after a regular manicure or pedicure if a salon's hygienic standards aren't up to par. And fake fingernails done in the best salon in town can harbor infection if not touched up every two weeks. The most important thing to remember (and something any good nail technician will stress when you have them applied for the first time): Fake nails are not low-maintenance; they require a commitment of money and time. Even though nail color itself lasts much longer on a set of wraps or tips—although most technicians still suggest you reapply a top coat every few days— you must commit to going to the salon every two weeks to have a refill or touch-up. If you don't have the money or the time for the upkeep fake nails require, don't get them.

What every first-timer should also know is that removing wraps and tips is less than fun. In fact, the first time you have tips removed, you realize why so many women keep theirs on. After the nail polish has been removed, you have to keep your fingertips dipped in a special solvent (which is essentially a really strong nail polish remover—smell and all) for up to 15 minutes. The nail technician then takes an orange stick or a metal cuticle pusher and begins to loosen the material from your natural nail bed. This process, especially when done by a bad technician, puts a lot of pressure on the natural nail. Clippers should never be used to remove acrylic nails—it damages the nail plate—and you should not try to remove them yourself at home.

And finally, what most women know but refuse to admit: No matter what anyone tells you, fake nails almost always look fake. There is really no way around it. Due to the thickness of the nail with acrylic or wraps on it, it is virtually impossible to recreate a natural-looking fake nail. There is no shame in this; just don't fool yourself.

Fake nails at home

There are kits you can buy at drugstores and beauty supply stores that allow you to give yourself a set of fake talons. A word to the wise, though: They are not easy to use. If a nail polish brush gives you trouble when all you are doing is applying color, it is probably not a good idea to attempt to give yourself a set of extra-long fake nails at home.

Post-Manicure **Hand Care**

INCORPORATE THE FOLLOWING ELEMENTS INTO YOUR BEAUTY ROUtine for just one week. You will notice a difference in your hands immediately.
• Push cuticles back with the edge of your towel after a shower.
• Each day, apply an SPF-formula hand cream that blocks UVA and UVB rays to protect against aging. Hand cream also helps to keep ashiness at bay.
• Touching up chips with the original nail color and a top coat application, also *vale la pena*. You can ensure yourself an entire week of beautiful nails this way.

En La Casa Foot Care

1) Remove polish.
Begin by removing old nail polish from your toes. The technique explained earlier for the fingernails is especially important for the toenails if you are removing a dark color to apply a lighter one. The technique removes color effectively, something you'll appreciate when doubled over trying to rid the cuticle area of the last vestiges of red toenail polish.

2) Clip or file the nails.
If you have been keeping up regular pedicures, there should be no reason to

Mami **says:** "A woman's true age is revealed by her hands."
Doctor says: Forewarned is forearmed. "Unless you wear *guantes* every day, you will definitely develop wrinkles on your hands; and the less pigment you have, the more your skin will be damaged. It will get very thin and bruise easily," says Houston dermatologist C. Enrique Batres, M.D. The hands are the part of the body that takes the most abuse, and they are exposed to sunlight year-round. Dr. Batres recommends using a daily sunscreen that contains an SPF of 15 or higher.

Beauty myth **busted!**

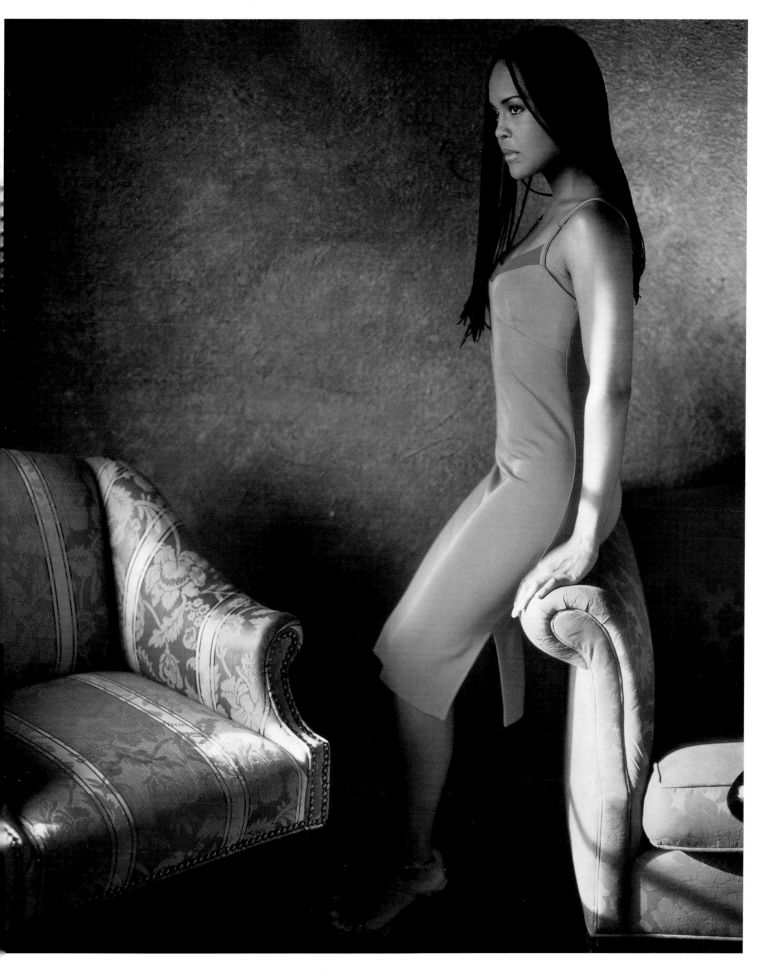

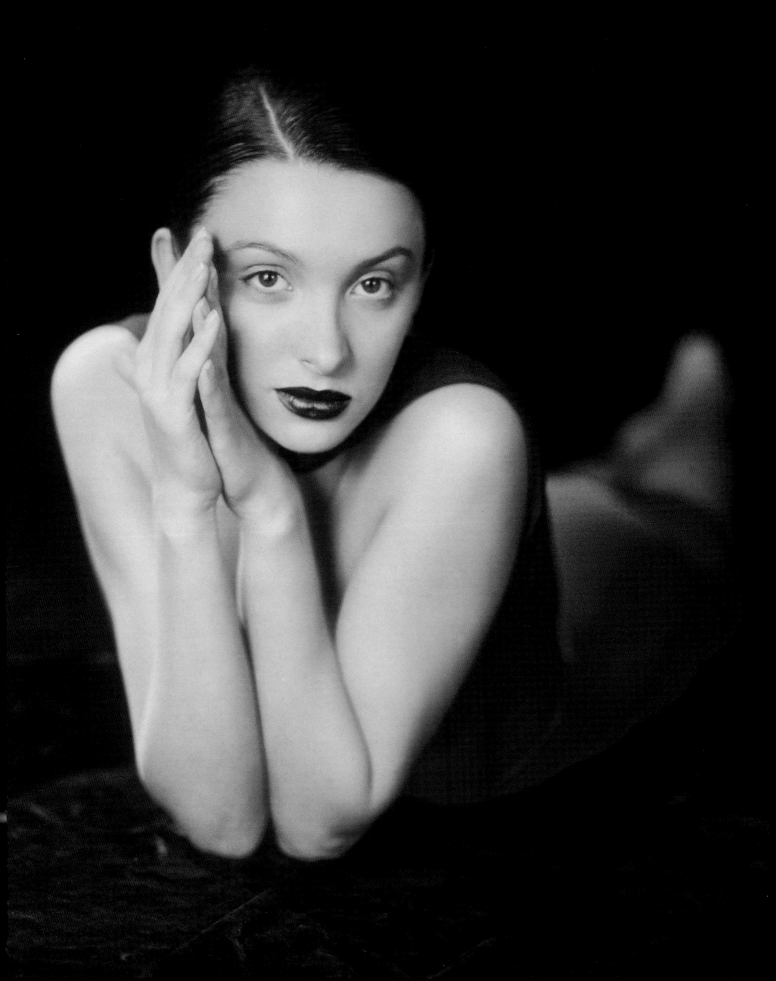

A course-grain nail file (right) for the toes. Fine- and course-grained foot files (below) for the feet.

have to clip your toenails. Toenails grow at a slower rate than the fingernails, and the toenails should be at a manageable length where filing with a medium-to-coarse emery board for natural nails should be enough. File and shape the nails straight across. Filing them too far down on the corners could result in an awful ingrown toenail that's painful to look at let alone have. If you must clip your toenails, do so to the length desired. Clip straight across, leaving the corners alone.

3) File the feet.

Before plunging ahead into the footbath, take out the foot files. Some foot files are double sided, with course and fine grain sides. Start with the coarse side of the file and concentrate on the areas prone to developing calluses: the tops of toes, the ball of the foot, and the heel. Go gently with the coarse side, since overfiling can lead to increased sensitivity on these areas. Most coarse files will leave the surface of the skin quite rough, so you want to follow with the fine-grain file. A good fine-grain file will leave the skin smooth and soft. A fine-grain file can also be used for areas of the feet (especially toes) that may be too sensitive for the harder, coarser file.

Some women prefer pumice stones to files. The major difference between pumice and files is that pumice stones should be used on wet feet, during the footbath or in the shower, while files are used on dry skin. The advantage of files over pumice is that they have specific, varying degrees of roughness. Plus, because you are using them on dry feet, you can more easily target smaller trouble spots like the top side of your end toes that are prone to developing calluses. The best of both worlds is to keep a pumice in the shower and give your feet a quick rubdown once a week, and then every two to three weeks do the more heavy-duty filing required for a pedicure.

Pedicure tools to avoid are the implements that use razor blades. Regular rubdowns with the pumice or filing eliminates the need to resort to the razor; there are, quite simply, too many accidents that can happen to the skin if you use the blade. Avoid using that at the nail salon, as well. Just because it's an esthetician wielding the blade doesn't make it any safer.

4) Give yourself a footbath.

The next step is the best part of a pedicure: the footbath. You can easily do a simple soap-and-water routine, but if you have the time, give yourself a more sensual footbath by adding essential oils to the water. Simply fill a tub with very hot water; add soap and a few drops of your favorite oil, such

Lujoso vs. bueno, bonito, y barato

THE TOOLS FOR AN AT-HOME PEDICURE CAN be purchased at beauty supply stores or drugstores:

Splurge
- foot file (one with a coarse and fine side, or two separate files—one fine, one coarse)
- nail file (coarse grain, but still for natural nails)
- rich foot cream
- cuticle cream
- pumice cuticle pusher

Save
- nail brush
- orange stick to clean the nail
- toe separaters
- base coat
- color
- top coat

Simple, sheer nails on hands and feet are both sexy and elegant.

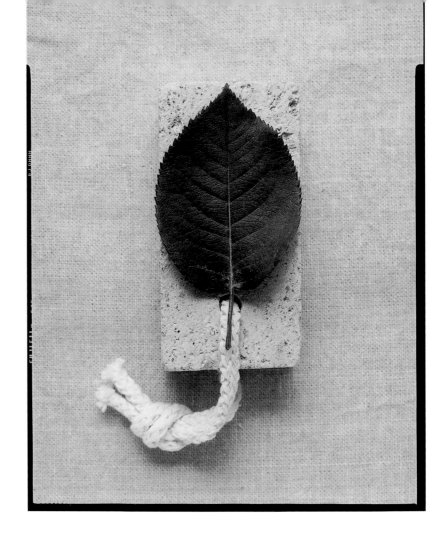

A pumice stone (right) provides a natural way to slough off dead skin. Below, have fun while you indulge in a footbath.

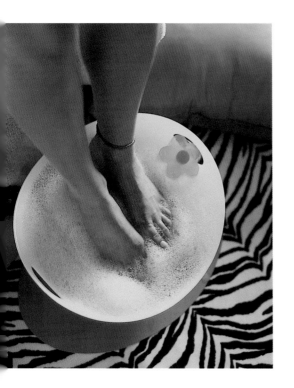

as lemon, mint, or rosemary. A foot bath is meant to clean the foot—not leave it prunelike—so after letting the feet soak for about five minutes, take the nail brush, douse it with soap, and scrub away, cleaning under the nails and between the toes. If you have a brisk, firm nailbrush, also scrub the feet themselves, to exfoliate the skin on the feet one last time. (Filing or using a pumice stone has the same effect, so if you have used a file already, go easy with the brush.)

5) Push back the cuticles.

After you are done with the bath, dry your feet with a soft towel. Apply cuticle cream to the toes. Gently use the end of the orange stick to loosen any debris from under the toenails and along the edge of the nail and cuticle. If you have cuticles that need pushing back, use the pumice. Do not cut the cuticles. Only trim large hangnails.

6) Give yourself a foot massage.

Here's where the pedicure gets sexy: Take the time to give yourself a luxurious foot massage with a generous application of rich foot cream. Massage the feet using your fingers, especially the thumbs. Move them in a circular motion over the tops of the feet and toes, up to the ankles. For each toe, gently rotate the digit in circular movements, After you have rotated each toe, rotate the entire front part of the foot, keeping the heel of the foot steady.

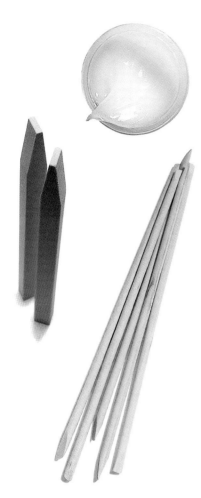

Tools for the hands are similar to those for the feet, with a few extras: Cuticle cream, pumice cuticle pushers, and wood sticks (above), enhanced by an extra rich foot cream (right), which you can slather on while giving yourself a foot massage.

Mami says: "Don't cut your cuticles. It's bad for your nails."
Manicurist says: *Mami*'s right. Cutting off too much cuticle irritates the nail and causes the skin to grow back thicker. It also causes annoying hangnails. Keep cuticles healthy by regularly pushing them back with the edge of a towel after you shower.

Beauty myth **busted!**

7) Prepare for color.

Remove excess lotion from the base of the nail (using nail polish remover, just as you did on your fingernails) to prepare the nails for polish. Take out the toe separators and lace one between each toe on each foot. Toe separaters make a big difference when you are giving yourself a pedicure. Since you are twisted up into a yoga-type position for the entire pedicure, anything that makes your polish aim a little better is worth it.

8) Apply the enamels.

Apply the base coat to each nail. Follow with the color in the same way described for the hands. Be especially careful to control the amount of polish applied to the smaller toes.

Post-Pedicure **Foot Care**

WHILE A PEDICURE LASTS TWO TO THREE WEEKS, GIVING YOUR FEET only that amount of attention is simply not enough. Feet require regular care.

● Applying a foot cream to your feet every night before bed makes a big difference in the appearance of corns on the toes. Try it for just one week. You'll see the difference.

● If you don't mind the slightly damp feeling you get, you can also put on a pair of cotton socks at night after you have applied the cream. This is akin to a deep-conditioning treatment for your feet.

● Wearing shoes that don't rub against the tops of the toes also makes a huge difference. Ultrahigh, pointy-toed heels look sexy, but if they hurt your feet and leave you with a corn that lasts a lot longer than the one season the shoes were in, are they worth it?

● If you have problems with very rough areas of the foot, consider using a rich foot cream or moisturizer that contains alpha hydroxy, beta hydroxy, or salicylic acids in the formula. These will exfoliate the surface of the skin while still providing moisture.

● Cleaning your feet in the shower with an antibacterial soap will help combat foot odor. Make sure the soap contains an ingredient that kills odor-causing bacteria for up to six hours.

● Avoid purchasing plastic shoes. Plastic does not allow the foot to breathe and can lead to awful, smelly feet. This is especially true in the summer months, since a lot of sandals are now being made with plastic instead of leather. Women think that since sandals have straps instead of fully encasing the feet, the smell won't be an issue. Wrong.

When it comes to the feet, adornment doesn't stop with the toenails. Feet are incredibly sexy and beautiful—be proud of a pair of pretty feet. Don't stop at toe rings, either. Experiment with menhdi (henna-based temporary tattoos), body paints to draw designs on your foot, adhesive body jewels, or even toenails with tiny designs. Especially if you work in an uptight, closed-toe-shoe corporate environment, where even the sight of a woman's toes is considered too casual, you have nothing to lose; the only people who will see your fabulous toenail designs are the people you choose to show them to outside the office.

How to Spot a
Quality Nail Salon

AS WITH ALL BEAUTY SERVICES, THE BEST WAY TO FIND A GOOD salon is through a recommendation. If you can't get a good recommendation, go and check out a place before you book an appointment. You are there to assess the salon's hygienic practices. Every nail station should have equipment to sterilize tools, and each new manicure and pedicure should begin with a fresh set of sterilized tools.

Do not be shy about insisting your own set of tools be used for a manicure or pedicure. A salon that has a regular customer base, an essential sign of any good nail spot, may even have a special area where they keep each regular customer's set of tools. Bringing your own tools is also the only way to ensure against the risk of fungal infection. Even the best salon in the world gets a few clients who may be unaware that they have toe fungus, and all it takes is a nail technician to neglect to sterilize her tools properly for the infection to spread to the next client. But any salon that cares about its clientele will gladly accommodate your preference that your own implements be used.

The best thing about beautifying your feet and nails: Ultimately, they are the lowest-maintenance areas of the body. With a once-a-week manicure and once-every-two-weeks pedicure, you won't have to think about your hands and feet for the rest of the time.

Maestro minuto

HAIR ON THE TOES AND FEET ARE COMMON for many women. The best method for removal, according to New York City manicurist/pedicurist Mary Hernandez, is to wax the hair from the root. Shaving the hair may seem like an immediate solution but only results in unattractive stubble, Hernandez says, which is particularly noticeable if you are fair-skinned.

Nail no-go's

• LONG, OVERGROWN TOENAILS, NO MATTER how pedicured they are or how many designs you have on them, look like switchblades. Playing footsie with a loved one can turn dangerous. Maintain toenails at a normal, healthy length. If you can't see the top of each toe above the edge of each nail, your toenails are too long.

• Do you want people to notice you or your nails? If it's the latter, then keep growing them excessively or get tips that make people wonder how you do things like take out your contacts without gouging your eye or answer the phone without breaking a nail. When words like "interesting" and "very long" are used to describe your nails, you will know you have succeeded in drawing all attention away from you and delivering it to your fingernails. Let attention be paid where it is due; you deserve to be front and center, not your nails, mama. Cut those too-long fingernails.

• Don't leave the rest of your nails long when one (or worse, more) is broken. It's silly and looks terrible. No one looks at your hands and thinks, Oh, what pretty, long nails. They look at your hands and think, Oh, she has four long nails and one short, stubby one. If you really can't stand to trim them, pay a manicurist who can give you a wrap or a tip while the broken nail grows out.

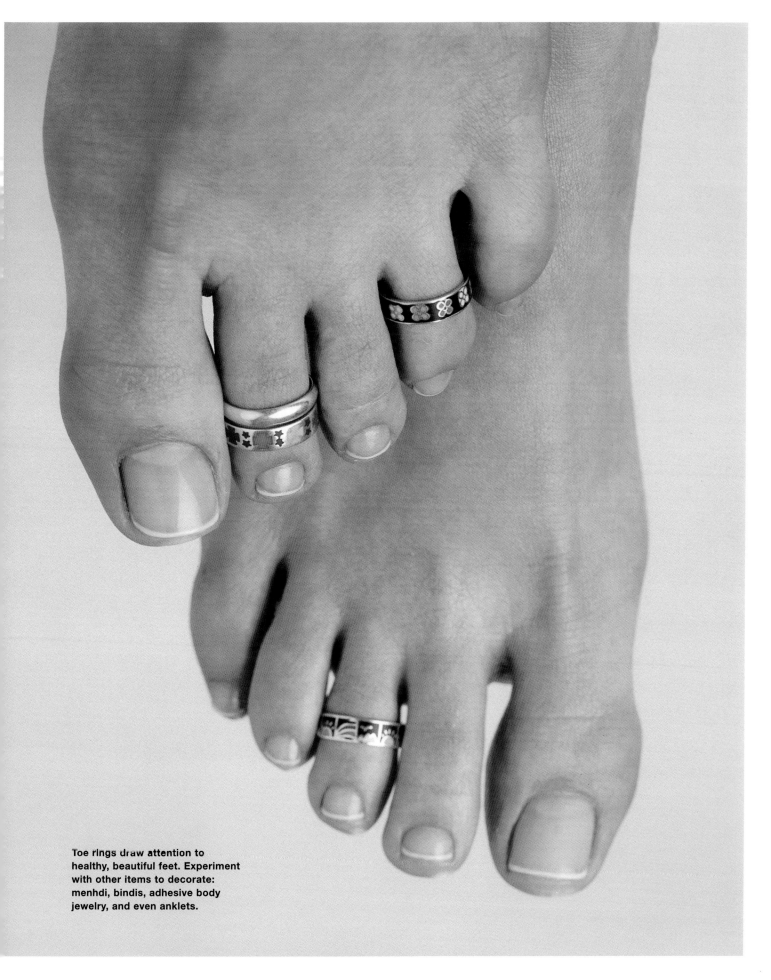

Toe rings draw attention to
healthy, beautiful feet. Experiment
with other items to decorate:
menhdi, bindis, adhesive body
jewelry, and even anklets.

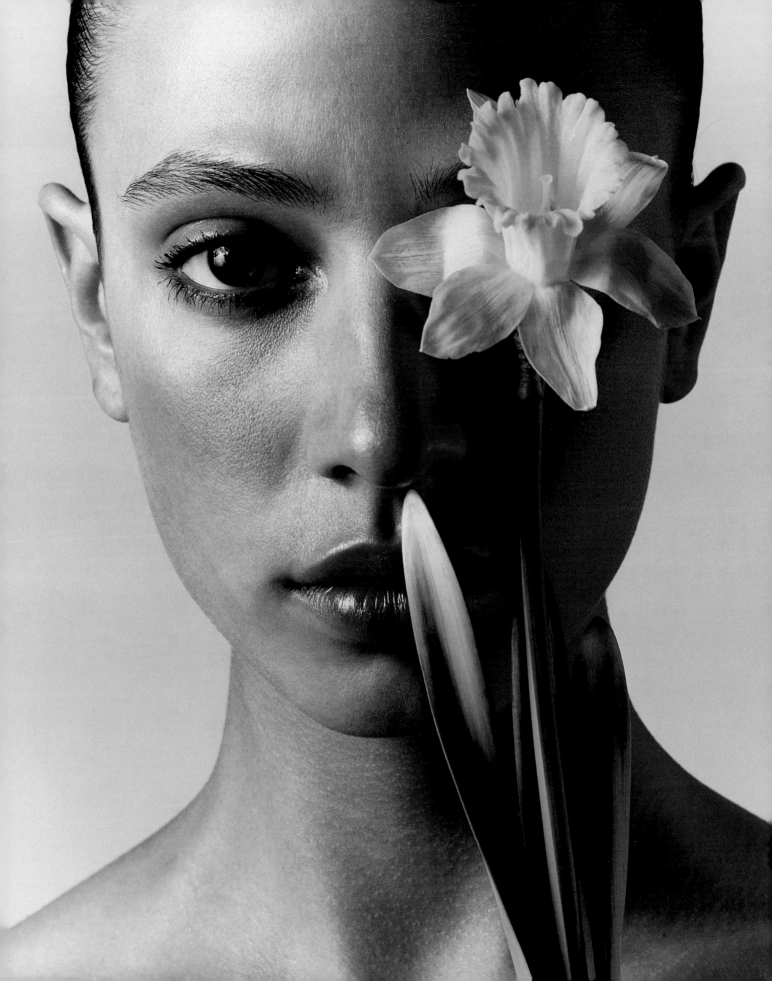

Scent-*ido*

FRAGRANCE HAS BEEN FREED FROM THE PERFUME BOTTLE. IT'S LIKE A GENIE THAT CAN be unleashed whenever you desire, one that can help lift your mood, change your mindset, or indulge your feelings. Scents are no longer limited to your mama's "signature" fragrance—the one she always applies before leaving home. Scents have now established their place in our homes and in our baths as well as on our bodies.

What incense does for the inside of a church, a fragrance can do for you. It creates an impression, shifts a mood, and leaves an indelible memory.

Making sense of all the fragrance hoopla is another story. Words used to describe a scent always fall short; it's like trying to define the complex, rich flavor of your favorite *flan* to somebody who has eaten only vanilla pudding pops. But once you know the language and connect the types of scents to the words, it becomes easier to describe the elusive properties of the fragrances you love.

What Makes a **Scent**

A SINGLE FRAGRANCE CAN BE COMPOSED OF A MULTITUDE OF SCENTS. Fragrances are not static. They change over time and "develop" by responding to the body chemistry of the person who has it on, as well as to environmental factors like temperature.

Each fragrance is composed, like a piece of music, by top, middle, and bottom notes. The top note is defined as the first impact or impression that a scent has—the note you smell immediately upon opening the bottle or applying it to your skin. Top notes last around 15 minutes, after which you can begin to detect the middle notes, which last up to an hour. It is from the middle notes that a fragrance is defined as being a certain type, such as citrus or floral. Middle notes become, in essence, the fragrance's identity. The bottom notes of a fragrance are what people are remarking on when they tell you how great you smell hours after you have applied your fragrance. In general, the fragrance you buy at the department store contains from 9 to 15 distinct notes.

Given the composition of a fragrance, it's understandable why many women make the mistake of purchasing one based on its first impression, or judging from the top notes only. This brings up one of the most important tips regarding fragrance: Try before you buy. Apply a fragrance where you normally would and see how the scent wears on you throughout the day. Rubbing your wrist against a fragrance sampler (the kind that comes in magazines) isn't a substitute for the real thing, since these samples can only recreate the chemical composition of a scent. You won't know how the actual fragrance reacts to your body chemistry until you wear the formula.

The other reason to try it firsthand is that even highly popular, instantly recognizable scents smell slightly different on different people. Your own body chemistry affects how a fragrance will smell. Oily skin, for example, tends to "hold" scents better and longer than dry skin. Heat and perspiration can also heighten the impact of a fragrance, one reason women are advised not to apply a scent before spending a day in the sun. Also, the high-fat, spicy diet traditional in our culture makes fragrances react more intensely with our body chemistry. These factors suggest that if you have oily skin, live in Texas, and eat lots of jalapeños and refried beans, you need to go easy with the atomizer, or people will smell you before they see you.

"A Latina is not ashamed to be a woman. She rejoices in being a woman, and celebrates her womanliness—being affectionate, loving men, not ever being ashamed to feel emotions. We should not lose our expressiveness, our love of life, our love of romance and sex and living."
—MIRIAM COLÓN

Your menstrual cycle affects how you may perceive a scent. In the first half of your cycle, your sense of smell is heightened, making you more aware of a fragrance's subtle notes. Pregnancy can also heighten your sense of smell—as anyone who has suffered from morning sickness can tell you. It's not uncommon for a pregnant woman to develop an intolerance to fragrances (and odors in general) that were pleasant to her when she was not pregnant.

Types of scents

Woodsy

Crisp, distinct scents that immediately evoke the forest and out-of-doors. Examples are sandalwood, oak, cedar, fir.

Citrus

Sharp fruit, tangy and refreshing scent; bergamot, lemon, orange, tangerine, lime, grapefruit. Citrus scents are used as top notes in many fragrances.

Floral

Flower-based scents, the easiest to identify and most common; rose, gardenia, freesia, lavender, jasmine, carnation, lilac.

Musk

Originally derived from animal scents, musks are often referred to as having "animal-like" notes. Current chemical reproductions mimic these scents identically. Often used as base notes, typical examples include patchouli, musk, civet, ambergris, castoreum.

Herbal

These notes can be spicy or sweet, like the herbs themselves; cardamom, thyme, rosemary, marjoram, sage.

Green

Think of freshly cut grass or dewy leaves. Green notes are often used as top notes of a fragrance. Grass is the most common of the class.

Mint

Scents that are easy to recognize; peppermint, spearmint.

Camphor

Think of your mother's cure-all, Vicks VapoRub, and you will know this scent immediately. Some Hispanics believe that placing a piece of camphor in a vessel of water helps to draw negative energies from the environment.

Here are some suggestions on picking a type of scent to fit your mood. While these are by no means hard-and-fast rules, they can help you figure out what to look for.

Energetic—green, spicy, and woodsy scents.

Relaxed—single florals and fruity blends.

Romantic—a floral bouquet.

Erotic—musky blends.

Fragrancia in the fridge

IN THE QUEST FOR FRESH FRAGRANCES AND frugal finances, some *muchachas* store their favorite scents in the refrigerator in an effort to help them last longer. This does work with eau de parfum and eau de toilette, but keep your perfume on the shelf. Since perfumes are a purer mix of essential oils, extreme cold temperature will upset the more volatile balance. Outside of the fridge, most fragrances will last one year.

Body

ENVELOPING YOUR BODY IN A SCENT IS THE MOST FAMILIAR, HIGHLY personal way to use fragrance. It's like creating an aura for you that everyone can sense, even if they can't see it.

Fragrances are variously defined, but the easiest way to approach them is according to their strengths. This gives you a better idea of what you are applying, how it will affect your "fragrance aura," and what you can add to it as the day goes on.

While generalizations can be made regarding a formulation's theoretical potency, it is pertinent to note, again, that due to individual body chemistry, skin type, and temperature, the same amount of eau de parfum on the same pulse point lasts different lengths of time on different people. Most fragrances are a blend of the pure fragrance—essential oils that create the scent—and a certain amount of alcohol. In any case, here are the most frequent types of fragrances you will find at the cosmetics counter:

Botanica in the **barrio**: A strong belief in the power of scent is part of our culture. Some perfumes are thought to contain special properties that can bring love, money, good luck, or health to the wearer.

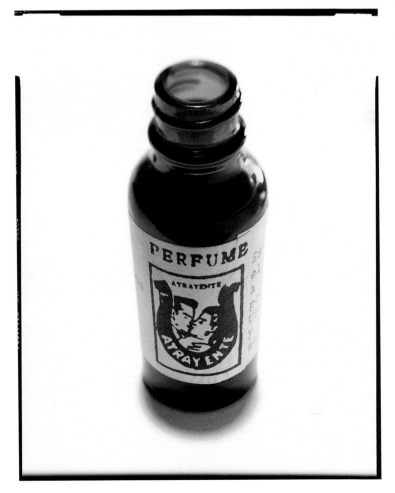

Perfume

The most concentrated formulation. Around 20 percent essential oils; lasts four to six hours. Perfume is more effective when applied with an atomizer than with the fingers; the spraying action diffuses the alcohol and permits the pure fragrance to adhere to the skin.

Eau de parfum

10 percent essential oils; lasts four to five hours. When "layering" fragrance—enhancing it by using different products with the same scent—eau de parfum can be used as a base.

Eau de toilette

5 percent essential oils; lasts two to four hours.

Eau fraîche

3 percent essential oils; lasts two hours. This is also commonly called a body splash and is meant to be applied immediately after bathing.

Cologne

2–3 percent essential oils; lasts two hours. This is the lightest form of fragrance. You can be more generous with your application since the scent is short-lived. Cologne can also double as an environmental fragrance when sprayed on linens and curtains. Fragrances with a high

Did you **know?** Latinas are twice as likely as non-Hispanic women to use fragrance every day.

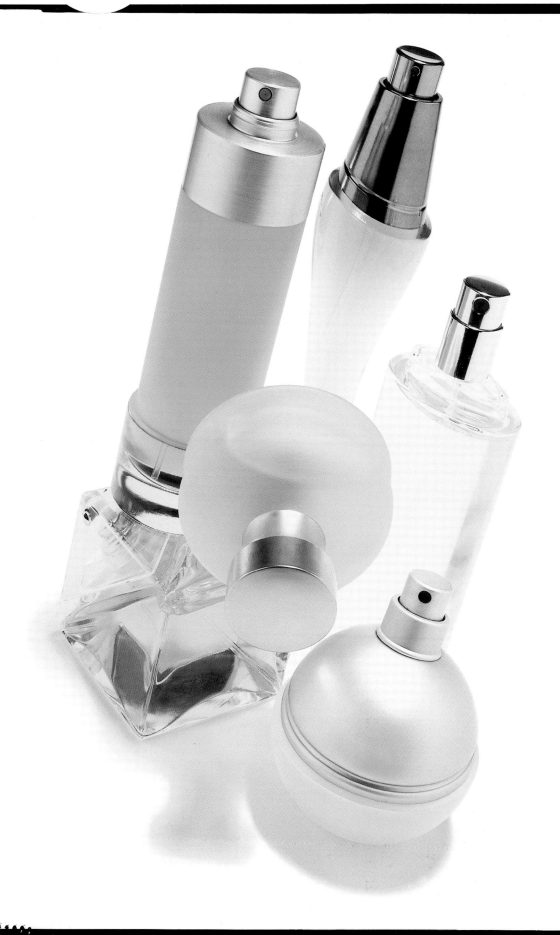

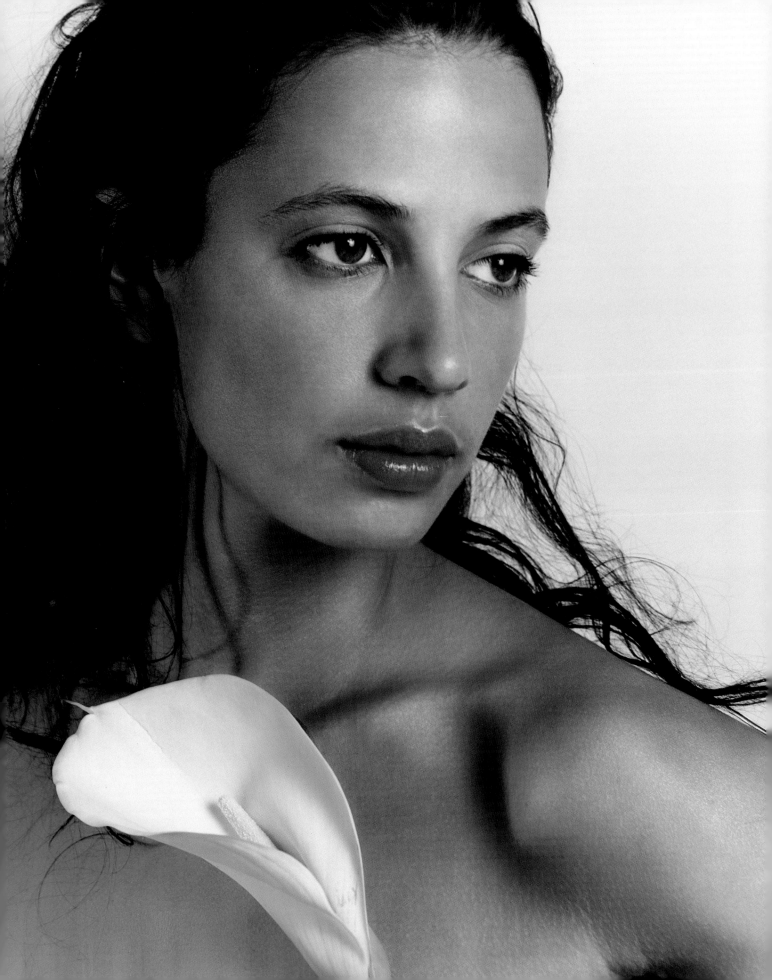

alcohol content evaporate quickly and can be spot-applied to certain areas of the body where you want a quick, refreshing boost: feet, hands, nape of the neck, etc.

Body mist

Potency depends on formulation, but generally lasts no longer than cologne. A newer evolution of body fragrances, mists contain a blend of light scent and moisturizers, making them great for the summer, when a heavy scent is unappealing and the formula's light moisturizers keep freshly bathed skin supple.

Perfume oils (for body)

Strong on initial application, the scent from perfume oils is not long-lasting because they contain no alcohol fixatives. Some women prefer their more natural, skin-soothing qualities.

Scented body lotion

5 percent essential oils; lasts three to eight hours, but overall effect is lighter than that of a liquid fragrance. Body lotion does double duty in that it moisturizes and scents the skin. Great to spot-apply to areas where you would normally apply lotion, although most do not—and are not meant to—have the moisturizing properties regular body lotions do. Scented body lotions are excellent for layering (see section below). If you have sensitive skin, body lotions with fragrance can be irritating, especially when you have just shaved or waxed the skin. Stick to regular lotion on these occasions.

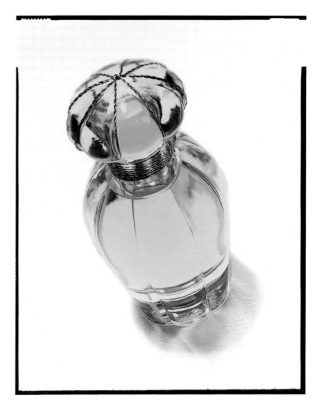

Fragrance began in the perfume bottle but now can be incorporated into our daily lives through a mix of methods.

Baño

BRINGING FRAGRANCE TO YOUR DAILY BATH HELPS YOU EXTEND THE indulgence of scent into yet another part of your life. As with regular fragrances, formulas have varying potencies that affect how you go about layering your scent.

Fizz bomb

Like Alka-Seltzer for your bathwater, these items bubble when submerged, and most release a fragrance. More fun than effective, the scent released by the fizz bomb won't last long.

Cologne

Try pouring some cologne or body splash into hot bathwater. The heat releases the fragrance, filling the bathroom and the water, surrounding you with the scent. The scent from this bath won't adhere to your skin, however, so it is not effective for layering.

Bath oil

Bath oil comes in many forms: foams, beads that dissolve when placed in hot water, and even bubbling bath oil. The resulting film that forms atop the bathwater adheres to the skin, softly coating the body in a *mantilla* of fragrance.

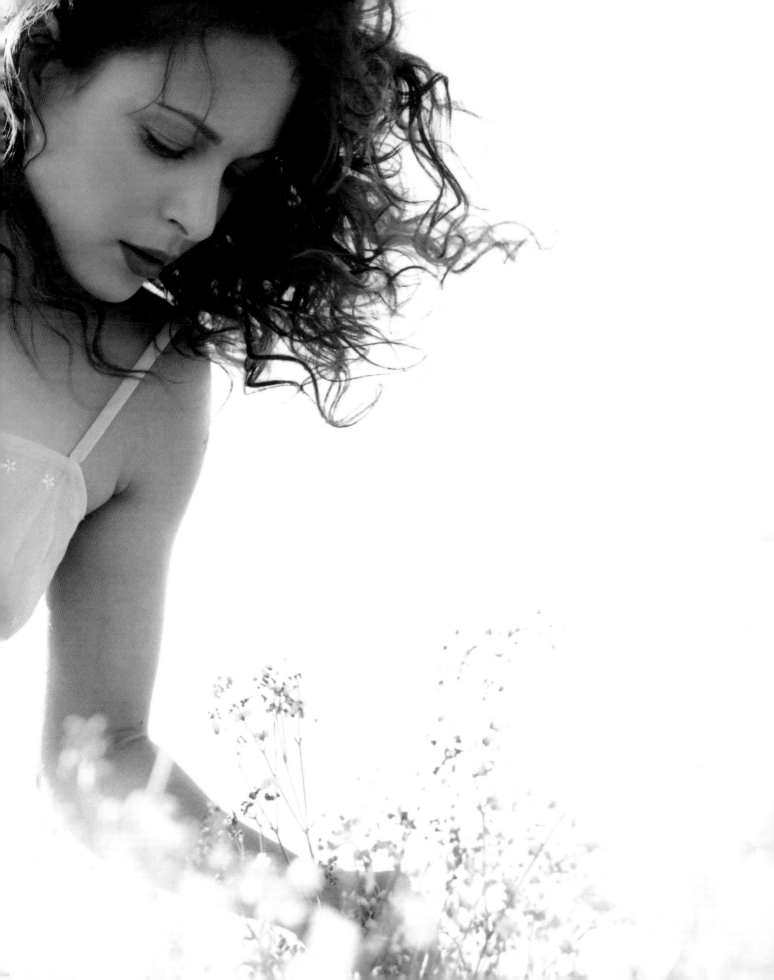

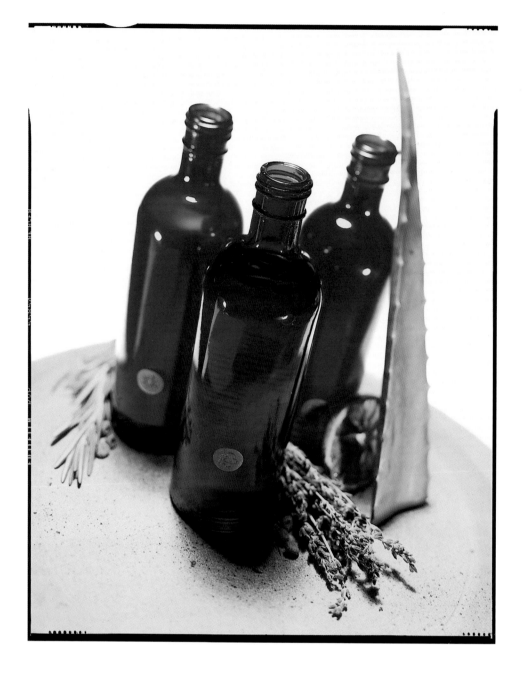

All fragrances are inspired by elements of nature. Even synthetic fragrances seek to mimic and capture the essence of rare or elusive plants, herbs, spices, and flowers.

Fragrance is more concentrated in bath oil, which means it will last longer on the skin. The oil also moisturizes the skin, heightening the pleasure factor.

Bubble baths

The most familiar way to add fragrance to your bath, bubble baths are made with a lot of detergents, which can be slightly drying to the skin, although many formulas are now made with conditioners. A bubble bath is more about relaxation and indulgence than anything else, since the fragrance does not last long on the skin once you leave the bath. One way to prolong the fun: Be sure not to add soap to the bathwater, even just by letting the bar fall into the water, as this causes the bubbles to evaporate.

Layering

THE SUREST WAY TO MAKE A SCENT LAST THROUGHOUT THE DAY IS to use different products with the same fragrance to "build" the scent around you. A typical layering process follows:

1) Indulge in a fragrant bath, using the bath oil or bubble bath version of your selected scent.

2) Slather on an application of lotion or body oil to spread the scent to the arms, legs, or wherever you need moisturizing.

3) Apply matching perfume or eau de parfum to pulse points; the inner wrists and the throat are the most common places.

Layering should be pure pleasure, not a chore. Do this when you have the time and the inclination; it needn't be part of your daily fragrance routine.

While layering makes the fragrance last throughout the day, you don't have to worry about being unable to shift gears and change moods for later in the evening. If you apply your scent early in the day, by the evening it will have run its course and you will be ready for something that matches your mood for the night.

Ambiente Aromas

OUR INDIGENOUS ANCESTORS USED TO BURN *COPAL* INCENSE FOR religious ceremonies. They knew the power fragrance has to change one's mindset and prepare, as *curandera* Elena Avila does, for worship. Today we have many means of bringing fragrance and its mood-enhancing benefits into our daily lives.

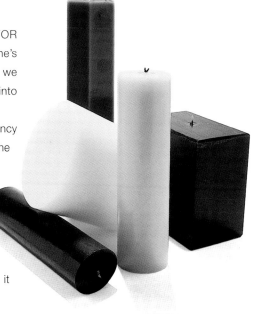

As with perfumes, purity and concentration of ingredients affect the potency of environmental fragrances. For long-lasting effect, you might find it worth the investment to buy high-quality environmental fragrances. If you want the option to change your room scent as the mood hits you, stick with the regular, cheaper versions.

Candles

The strongest-scented candles, made with fragrant oils, are also more expensive, but the difference they make in a room is enormous. The way to tell them apart in the store is relatively easy: When you touch the candle, it

"I go to my altar, I burn copal. I surround myself with the copal smoke and I actually pray out loud as if God were standing there right in front of me."
—ELENA AVILA

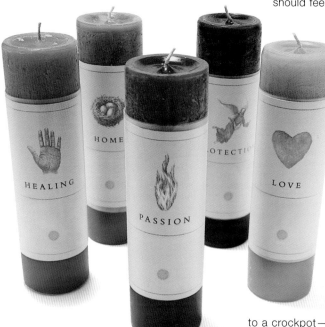

Candles and incense don't just produce fragrance, they create an entire ambience.

should feel more oily than waxy, the way a nonscented candle feels. Keep the fragrance strong by covering the candle (if it comes in a jar with a cover) when it is not lit and keeping the wick trimmed. Trimming the wick also helps prevent the candle from smoking and keeps burned wick from falling into the candlewax, which can lessen the impact of the fragrance.

Lightbulb oil rings

Generally made of metal, these coated rings release the fragrance of the oil when placed on a lit bulb. They are surprisingly potent and a great option for areas where a candle isn't suitable, such as an office space or anywhere children are present and an open flame would be a concern.

Potpourri

Potpourri consists of dried herbs, spices, petals, and flowers. The way to reap the greatest benefits from potpourri is to boil it in a pot on your stovetop. If you are a big fan of potpourri, you can purchase special potpourri warmers—similar to a crockpot—that use long-lasting low heat to keep the fragrance releasing continuously into the air.

Room sprays

An elegant take on (and redefinition of) the old aerosol air fresheners found in bathrooms, room sprays are now widely available at linen stores and any place home and bath items can be purchased. Simply spritz into the air and enjoy the scent. You can also make your own room spray by placing body splash in a spritzer and spraying on curtains, sofas or rugs; just make sure the items won't be stained.

Linen sprays

Linen sprays, only recently made widely available, are an excellent way to incorporate fragrance into daily life. Spray your linens either in the closet or directly on your bed, and at bedtime be welcomed by a wonderful fragrance. The linen sprays are formulated so that they won't stain or cause damage to the bedding. Aromatherapy blends that contain lavender or rosemary are said to have a calming effect and enhance sleep.

Incense

Sometimes referred to as mankind's original perfume, incense has been around since biblical times. Available in a range of scents, it can be used to evoke many moods but because of its smoke factor is generally used to set a sexy or spiritual tone. Opt for room sprays when you want freshness or an energizing jolt.

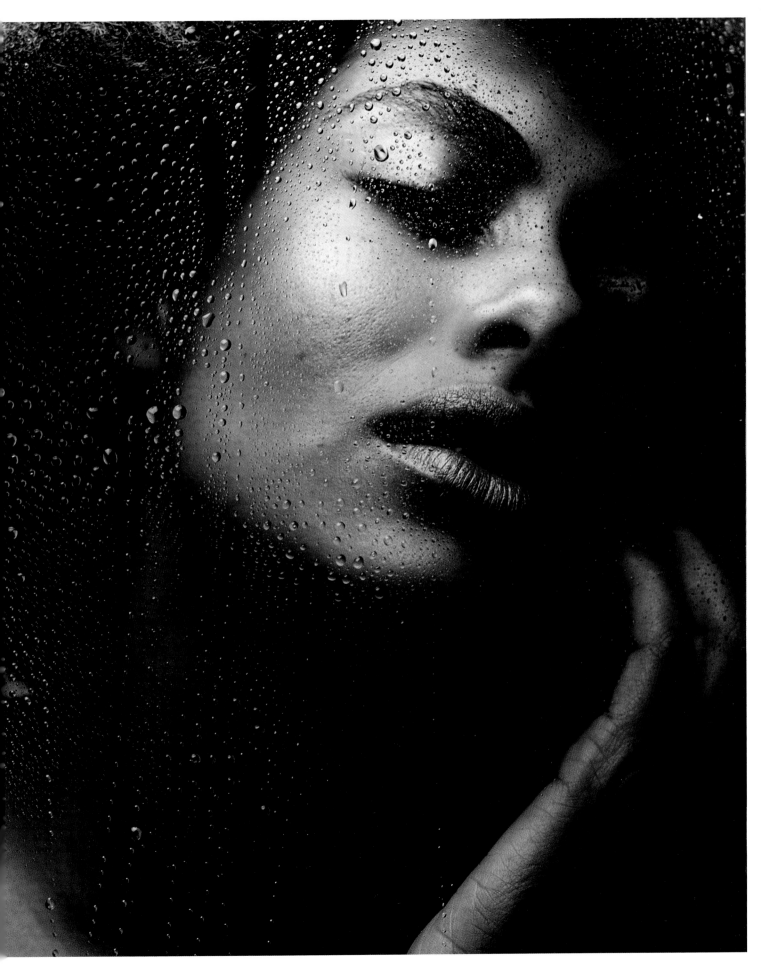

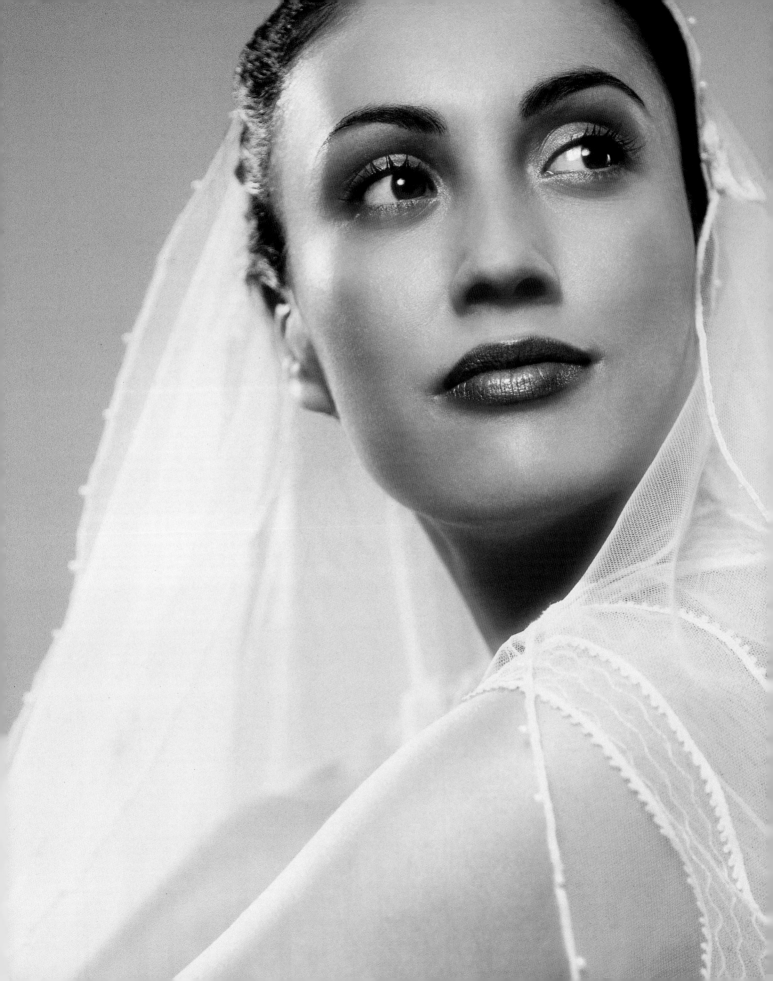

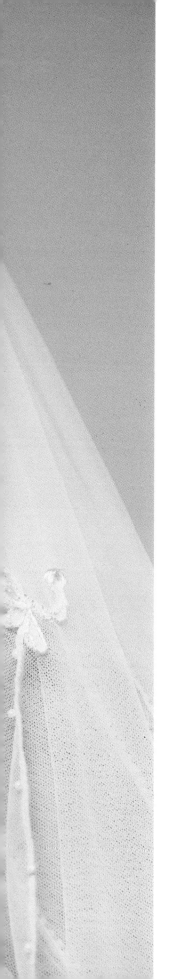

Celebrating Your Beauty:
Weddings and *Quinceañeras*

THE *MARIACHIS* ARE CONFIRMED. YOUR *TÍA LUPE* FINALLY fits into the two-sizes-too-small dress she bought six months too early so that she could look "petite" for the occasion. Your girl-friends have started dropping hints about the *escándalo* they'll be subjecting you to and the video camera they'll have on hand to capture every moment of the bachelorette party. Your mother has given you her series of "how to have *un buen matrimonio*" talks and has scheduled her appointment for the highlights she's having put in her hair.

Y tú? What about your needs for the big day? It's supposed to be about you and him—and his tux is rented—but are you ready?

When it comes to big-day beauty, it can be helpful to understand the many factors at work where your appearance is concerned. You want to look good for yourself and for the people who are there—everyone from the groom, who will be close enough to plant *el besote*, to the family and friends who have gathered to recognize and celebrate the importance of this occasion. You also want to look good for the photos and videos that will be taken to mark this special day in your life. In other words, you need to look spectacular close-up and breathlessly beautiful from a distance. The beauty mantra for the day is that you want people to notice *you*—not your nails or your hair or your makeup.

Even the pragmatic "I'm never getting married!" woman has high expectations for how she wants to look and feel on the day she breaks her *solterona-por-vida* pledge with the I'll-love-you-forever vow. Nasty little surprises like pimples, redness, heat, and rain, can show up to challenge the calm-and-cool, flawlessly serene demeanor you have labored to achieve. You also need makeup and hair that lasts—nothing that slides off the face after the first few hours. Sounds hard to pull off?

The solution is to be prepared: for the weather, for the nervous energy, and for the breakout and any other beauty-related mishap you can't control. If you can focus on being prepared instead of trying to be perfect, you will enter the church (and the photo-taking session, and the reception hall) with a lot more confidence.

Pre-**Wedding** and Pre-*Quinceañera* Beauty

MANY WOMEN MAKE THE MISTAKE OF DECIDING TO USE THEIR wedding or *quinceañera* or any big event as the chance to try every beauty procedure they have ever been remotely curious about. From tinting their eyelashes to getting a thong-ready Brazilian bikini wax to perming their hair, women who take a no-holds-barred approach to big-day beauty run the risk of winding up frizzy-haired, blotchy, broken out, and broke, since none of the procedures are cheap. It's fine to do some experimentation leading up to a major celebration, but you must do it with enough time to correct any mistakes. The key is to plan, and, if you can afford it, to give every procedure a trial run at least once before you commit to making it a part of your wedding day beauty regimen. This tactic has two benefits: You ensure that the procedure actually does what it is supposed to do, such as clearing your skin and making it glow instead of making you break out in hives; and if you decide not to opt for a procedure, you still have time to grow out its effects. Below are a list of the common things women decide to try before the big day as well as some beauty changes you should incorporate into your routine ASAP, along with a suggested time frame for implementing or testing each one.

Facials

If you insist on getting a facial even though you have never had one before, do the first one a month and a half before the wedding. After getting the facial, monitor your skin's reaction afterward—not only for the first few days but for the first two weeks, which is how long it can take if the point of the facial was to clear up any breakouts. If you liked the results, schedule a second one no closer than two weeks to a week and a half before the wedding, particularly if you are prone to breaking out or are very fair skinned and are having a pore extraction done. Facials can actually lead to acne, which many facialists say goes hand-in-hand with the excretion of impurities. Pore extractions, especially on sensitive or *güera* skin, can leave the area red for quite a few days. Plan accordingly so you don't have any surprises and can still enjoy the benefits of the procedure.

Eyelash tinting/perming

Eyelash tinting lasts a few weeks, while an eyelash perm can last up to three months. The idea behind getting these procedures done around a wedding is, of course, so that you are not left with a streaky face and straight, tiny stubs after tears of joy and the emotion of the day. It also has the bonus of giving you a great set of low-maintenance lashes for your honeymoon. A bit of what may seem like obvious advice: Don't have both procedures done at once. Decide what you need, then choose the appropriate treatment. Eyelash tinting is only useful for women with sparse, light lashes, whereas perming can give a great curl to *hermanas* with long, lush, black lashes that are, unfortunately, straight. As with the facial, do a trial run long before the wedding, so you can make an informed decision about having this done a week before the actual event. Also, some of these procedures are not available everywhere, either because some states do not allow them or because salon clients in the area never request them. Trying these out might involve some research on your part.

Bikini/eyebrow/lip wax

A lot of Latinas are already familiar with waxing and have it done on a regular basis. If this is true for you, stick with an esthetician who does this procedure to your satisfaction. This is not the time to go trying out new salons in town.

If you are trying one of these procedures for the first time, here are some things to remember: Even waxing done by the best esthetician can leave

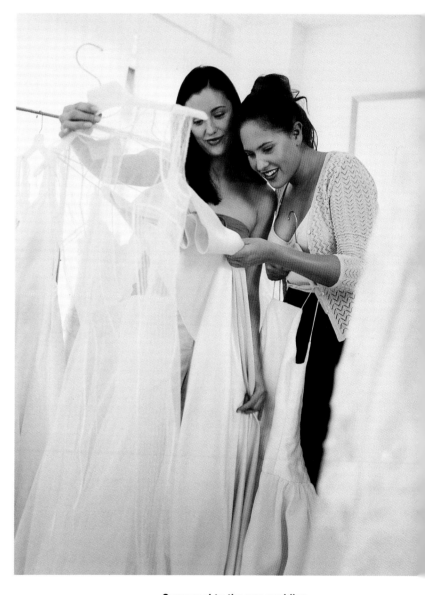

Compared to the pre-wedding beauty preparations some women subject themselves to, picking a dress is the easy part.

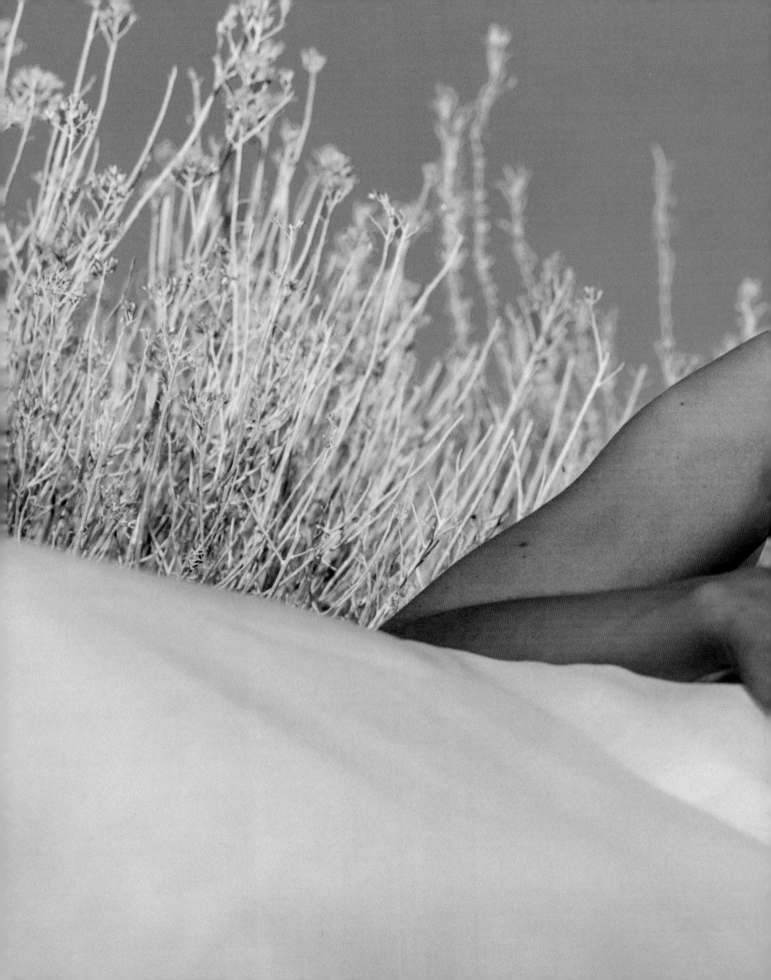

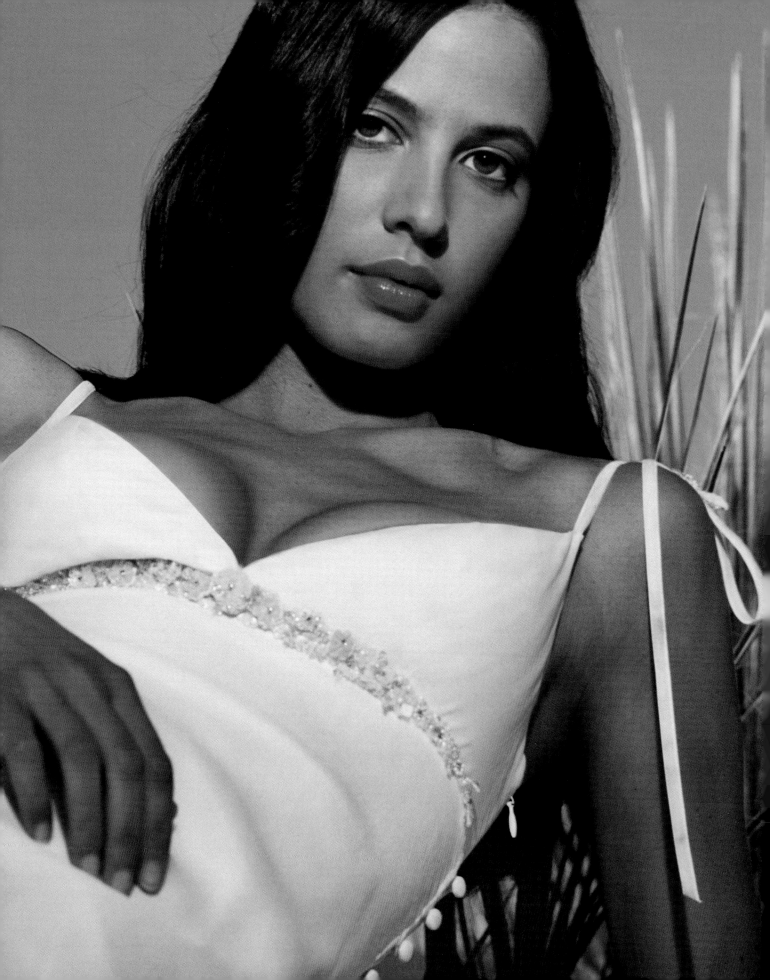

bumps, irritation, or redness on the skin, so have it done two full months before the event to see how your skin responds and whether the esthetician you use does a good job. Try to get a sense for how quickly your hair grows back. Then, one to two weeks before the big day, get the procedure done a second time.

The only exception to the above rule would be bikini waxes. Bikini waxes can be quite painful for first-timers, so be warned. Only go to an esthetician who has been referred to you. If you want to look good in your bridal thong, consider a Brazilian-style bikini wax, but again, do it with an esthetician you completely trust. Again, do not take aspirin before the waxing, because aspirin thins the blood, which can lead to increased bleeding and even bruising of the skin. Also, be aware of post-waxing skin care. Ingrown hairs can be avoided by exfoliating the bikini area daily or by the topical application of bikini line creams or astringents that prevent them. Depending on your hair regrowth cycle, a bikini wax can start to grow in after two to three weeks. If the window of time is shorter for you, schedule the final bikini wax a day or two before the ceremony—especially if you are going on a honeymoon where you will be on the beach.

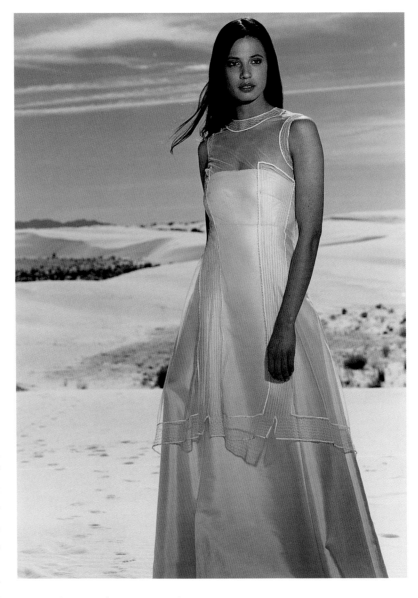

If facial waxing leaves you with a slight breakout in the area for a few days afterward, or if you tend to have acne-prone skin, skip the heavy creams some estheticians apply immediately after pulling the wax. Stick with an application of an astringent, such as witch hazel, instead. Later in the day, for extra protection, apply a layer of anti-acne cream on the waxed areas.

If you are trying to change the shape of your eyebrows for your wedding, give yourself ample time (at least six months) for the brow to be ready. Also, remember that eyebrow hairs do diminish with repeated removal from the root. You may be attempting to grow back a classical, slightly thicker brow for the wedding, only to find that it's a lot harder at 30 than when you were 20. Don't despair: A good makeup artist will teach you how to complete your look for the big day without appearing overly made up. In any case, attempts to change to brow shape should be done with plenty of time. Also, if you are waxing them for the first time, it's essential to experiment a few times before the big day. You want to have a shape you are happy with.

Artificial nails

Wraps and tips are one beauty indulgence that makes perfect sense for a wedding, although most estheticians would advise against it for 14-year-olds preparing for their *quinceañera*. The primary benefit is a manicure that lasts two weeks with little or no chipping. Since you have so many other things to worry about on that day, it can be a relief to have at least one thing absolutely in your favor.

Most important, if it is your first time, you should get a set of nails done two to three weeks before the big day so you can accustom yourself to how fake nails feel. They do take getting used to. You might also get a sense for how long you want your nails to be, although almost all nail estheticians will agree that, for the first time, shorter is better. If you feel comfortable and decide to keep the artificial nails for the wedding, the other benefit is that the next trip to the manicurist is simply for a fill—the application of acrylic or nail bonding material to the regrowth area at the base of the nail—and a polish change. The initial application is more time-consuming, at least 45 minutes. Fills should be done religiously every two weeks, so plan accordingly.

If it is your first time, go to a salon for which you have a reference from a friend. Make sure the place is immaculately hygienic; it would be awful to have your nails beautiful for the wedding, then end up with a fungal infection that takes a year to clear up. Tell the manicurist exactly how many eighth-inches or centimeters you want added to the nail. Being as specific as possible will help avoid misunderstandings. Remember that what may seem "short and functional" to an esthetician who is used to giving customers extremely long nails may seem awkward and unsightly to you. Tell her exactly what you want.

For color choices, keep nails simple, neutral, and sheer. Avoid designs, even if they are subtle.

Feet

If displaying perfectly manicured toes is part of your wedding day plan, then starting early is a must. Commit to regular pedicures once every two to three weeks without fail. Even more important than the pedicure, however, is the commitment to applying a rich cream to your feet at least three times a week, if not every night, before you go to bed. Throw out shoes that rub against your toes and present the risk of corns developing on your toes. If you have more serious problems, such as bunions or painful corns, see a podiatrist immediately. As soon as you select your shoes, gauge how much exposure your toes will be getting and take care of your feet accordingly. Get your final pedicure a few days before your wedding so you have one less thing to worry about the day before. As with the fingernails, avoid elaborate patterns or designs. Keep it simple. Bring your shoes with you to the pedicure, so you can make sure the toenail color selection fits.

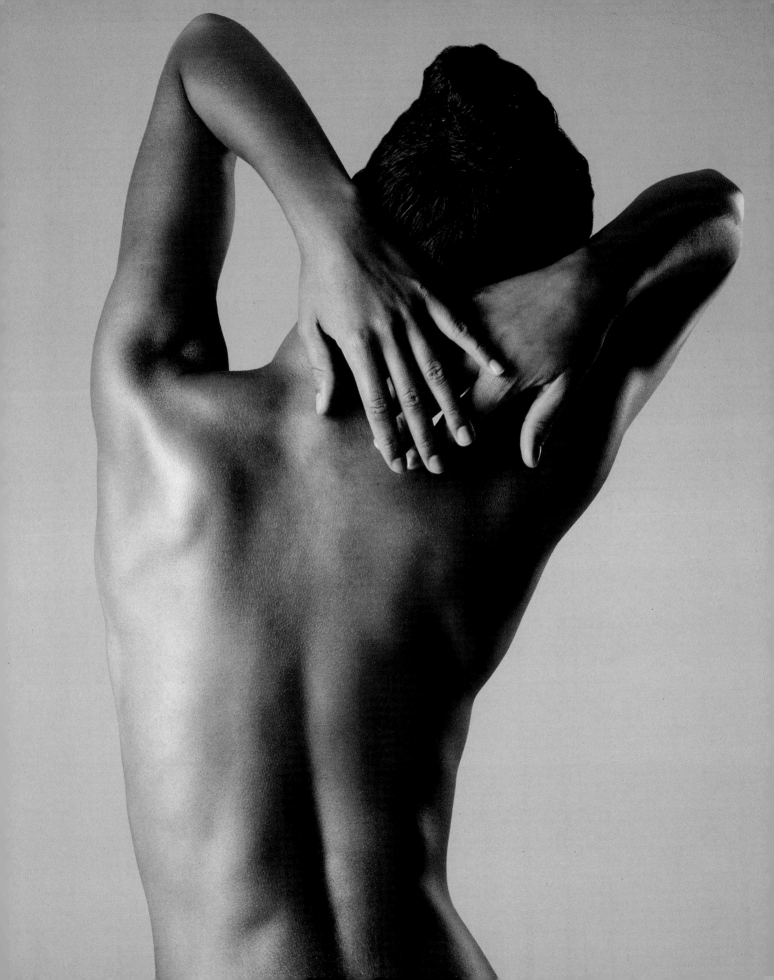

Tanning

Some women decide that on their wedding day, they should be not only gorgeous but bronzed. A lot of brides do this on the pretext that since they are going away for their honeymoon, they want to get a "base tan" so they can look good in a bikini. As you read in Chapter 6 ("Get the Glow"), tanning should really be done away with altogether, and a wedding is not the time to get the deep, dark, exotic tan you have maybe two months out of the year. Aside from the enormous long-term skin damage, tanning also tends not to look good in photographs, since skin does not tan evenly. It can also change your skin texture—not a smart idea, since you don't want to be dealing with surprises on the big day, whether it's dry, scaly skin or a breakout. Tans can also heighten skin discoloration or *manchas* acquired from too much sun exposure over the years.

Massage

One beauty treat you can leave for the day before: a full-body massage, to relax. You may also want to treat yourself (and your bridesmaids) to a full-body exfoliation. One note of caution: If you are getting a leg or bikini wax, never exfoliate immediately afterward. The skin is already raw and sensitive.

Hair changes

Hair changes are one of the best arguments for a long engagement. As anyone will tell you, a wedding or a *quinceañera* is not the time to try a dramatic new chemical treatment that will severely alter the health of your hair. Any experimenting should be done with a huge window of time so you can change whatever you don't like. Whether it's highlights or a body perm, really think about whether you need to have this done just before your big event. The best tactic is to stick with what you have, if you like it, or to talk with your hairdresser about making a subtle change.

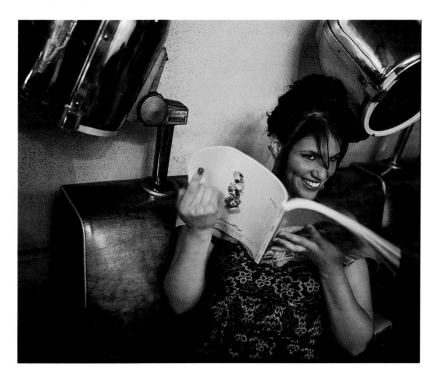

The place to experiment with different hairstyles is at the hair salon. This will help you make sure you look—and feel—your best when you make it to the altar.

That said, weddings can be a wonderful opportunity to try creating an updo with a hairpiece or—if you are willing to invest the money and time—natural-looking human-hair extensions. Without affecting the chemical composition of your hair, and thereby obviating any possible damage and the need for subsequent conditioning treatments, the right updo hairpiece can give you extra height and turn your *pelo* into a work of art on your big day. You should go to a specialist you absolutely trust, and, especially with the extensions, have them done at least two weeks before the ceremony. That way, you can get used to the change in length and experiment with how you want to style your new, long mane on the day of the event. Fake hair, like fake fingernails, takes getting used to, so the sooner you accustom yourself, the better.

The sweat factor

Most women don't worry about the sweat factor until a few days before the big event, when they realize that pure nerves could give them a glow—and not the glow of love. This is a mistake, primarily because the strongest antiperspirants do require some getting used to in terms of your body's production of sweat. If you normally use a deodorant without an antiperspirant, make the switch as soon as possible. In the weeks leading up to the *boda*, look for an antiperspirant with aluminum zirconium, the strongest commercially available ingredient, which is contained in some but not all antiperspirants. Check the label to make sure yours has it.

Also, take a tip from the armed forces. A week before long military exercises, soldiers begin prepping their feet with spray antiperspirant to reduce sweating and to protect against blisters and friction, leaving them callus- and blister-free. It sounds weird, and of course ideally you will have had time to break in the shoes by wearing them around the house. But barring that, a spray of antiperspirant can ensure a smooth walk, instead of a limp, down the aisle.

Selecting a makeup artist and hairstylist

This process should take place two to three months before the big day. By this time, you should have decided on a dress and a veil, as well as how long your hair will be on that day. These elements are necessary in order for your prospective makeup artist and hairstylist to recommend the most becoming look for the event.

As is so often the case, the best way to go about finding someone is through references. Talk to women whose weddings you have attended and whose makeup you loved. Or talk to women who regularly wear makeup well and see if they happened to learn their skills from one person in particular. If you have no way of getting personal references, the next best place to look is your local department store. Go to the counter that sells a cosmetic line you are familiar with and like, since makeup artists at these counters will be comfortable with those same products. If you still don't find someone you are pleased with, go to local salons. Many now offer makeup and hair services, which could make the entire process much easier for you.

Once you find a makeup artist you are willing to work with, ask to see a portfolio and insist on a test run. If the makeup artist seems to be resistant to doing this, find someone else immediately. The first time the two of you do makeup, make sure to bring photographs of what you want. Bring pictures from magazines, if it is helpful. This will help to ensure that both of you are talking about the same things. A good makeup artist will be honest with you about whether the photos you have brought are realistic in terms of your coloring or any changes you will make to your coloring by the wedding (mainly with your hair). Once you are sure both of you are on the same page, you can move forward with the actual makeup application.

The look most recommended for a wedding or a *quinceañera* is classical and beautiful, with neutral colors that will look good years from now. If the make-up artist starts by taking out the latest shimmery or glossy makeup colors— especially if you have oily skin—let him or her know immediately that looking "in" is not the goal on this day. Reflective and frosty makeup tends to look oily in photographs and should be avoided or, at most, applied sparingly.

Women who regularly use little makeup may leave a makeup artist's chair feeling as if a mask has been applied to their face. For the initial consultation, it is a good idea to come with your own makeup already on. This will give the makeup artist you are working with the clearest sense of how you look on a daily basis and how much more (or, in some cases, less) he or she will have to apply com-

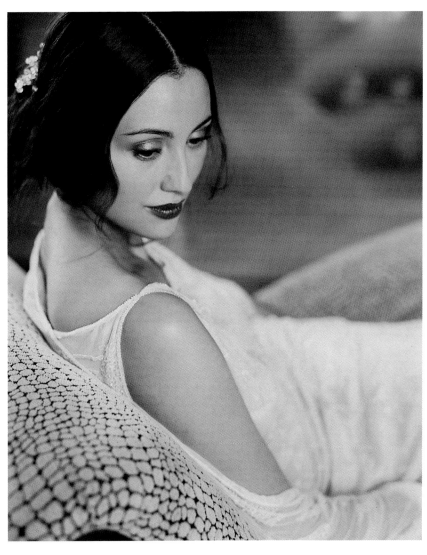

The uncomplicated, low bun on this bride matches her classical makeup. Both elements create the perfect compliment to the beautiful, elegant-yet-simple dress.

pared to what you are comfortable wearing. Be forewarned, though: While seeing how you normally use cosmetics may influence the makeup artist's choices, the effect she or he creates has to last the entire day and look good in photographs, so you will almost certainly be wearing more makeup than you customarily do.

It is also a good idea to bring photographs of yourself, particularly ones you like. This conveys a sense of how well you photograph to the makeup artist, who is not only trying to make you look fabulous to the people at the wedding but to the cameras recording the day. Let the makeup artist know what type of photography will be involved for the wedding—whether it is indoor or natural lighting, black and white or color, or some of each. Also let the makeup artist know if you will be sitting for portraits immediately after the ceremony or, as some couples now do, before the wedding or on a different day entirely. This will allow the makeup artist to supply you with a look that is easily touched up or to suggest a slightly different look involving more makeup or contouring techniques for the time you are sitting for portraits.

Remember that big-day beauty is all about details. If, for example, you are wearing a veil, you don't want to have thick, sticky, goopy gloss on your lips. God forbid you should get your veil stuck to your face as you walk down the aisle, and your *amorcito* has to kiss a face that has pink goo on the cheeks, chin—everywhere but the lips.

What you are looking for in a dry run, besides a beautifully made-up face, is:

• Makeup that will last hours

It may look beautiful when the artist first applies it, but what about four hours later? Are you shiny as a marble? Has the concealer around your eyes slid into the tiny wrinkles around your eyes? Be realistic about your expectations, however. Lipstick that stays on your lips after tearing through a plate of *chuletas* has yet to be invented. Also, if you tend toward exceedingly greasy skin, even the best makeup artist can't stop an oil spill.

• Makeup that looks like you, only better

The first person—and really, the only person—the makeup artist's handiwork should please is you. If the person working on you promises cheekbones where there are none, a full lip where a thin one lay before, and a few inches trimmed off your *papada*, then run, don't walk, the other way. These techniques sound good in theory, but unless they are done with the most expert application, they can end up making you look like a drag queen.

After you have had the makeup applied and decide you are fit to be seen in public, put the work to the test by looking at it in the different lights you will be under on the day of your wedding. If you are having an outdoor wedding, go outside. If it is an evening event, use this makeup job as an excuse to go out for the night and have fun, since that will hopefully be exactly what you will do on your big day anyway.

Once your face has passed the lighting test, run it by some real people. Do your friends and family recognize you? Do they look frightened at first sight of you, or amazed? If their reaction is the former, go find a new makeup artist. Most important, ask your *novio* to stand close to you and see what he thinks. Is he mesmerized by the vision of beauty before him, or is he seeking shelter from the mascara particles that fly everywhere with each blink of your overly made-up eyes? If it's the former, you and your makeup *maestro* are on the right track.

Hair help

In terms of your hair, you need to go to a hairstylist who is an expert hairdresser. Knowing what veil or *corona* you will wear and what your dress looks like is half the battle when it comes to a hair plan for the big event. Let your hairdresser know whether you will have the veil over your face as you walk into the church, and if it will be pulled away from your face for the remainder of the ceremony. These details are important because, in addition to pleasing you, what a good hairdresser will be concerned with is comfort, scale, and proportion.

Your hairdresser will have to know whether you are wearing a Princess-Di-meets-Scarlett-O'Hara-type dress or if you are going for a much more

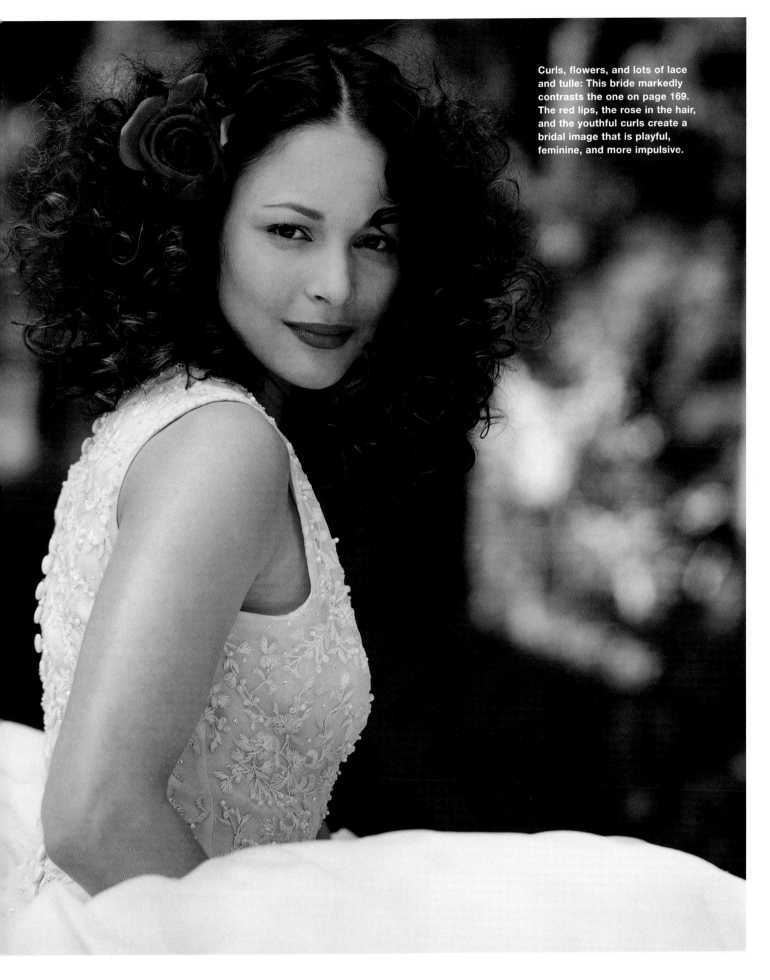

Curls, flowers, and lots of lace and tulle: This bride markedly contrasts the one on page 169. The red lips, the rose in the hair, and the youthful curls create a bridal image that is playful, feminine, and more impulsive.

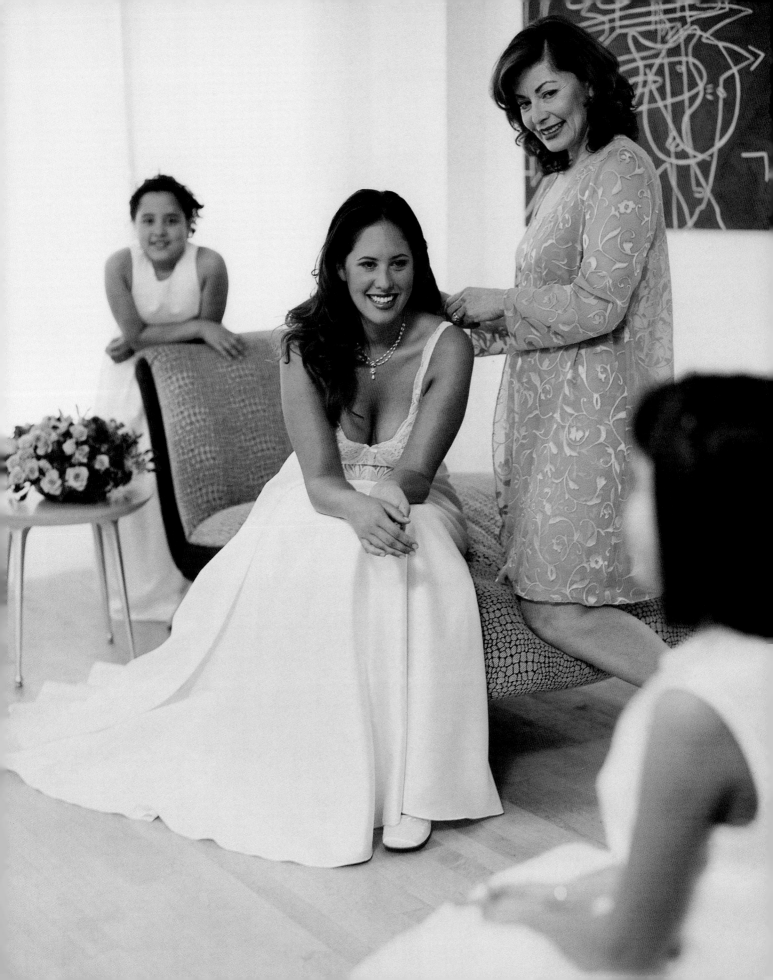

streamlined look à la the late Carolyn Bessette Kennedy. A good hairdresser will be ever mindful—and remindful—that on your big day, besides looking spectacular from every angle, you must look well proportioned, too. As we eye ourselves in the mirror, women tend to forget that the rest of the world sees us from top to bottom, front to back, side to side. So your hairdresser must have panoramic vision—and share it with you. Like your makeup, the hairstyle and headpiece will require a dry run to test how they'll hold up for the day. We have all experienced the horrors of curls gone limp, hair turned frizzy, or a nasty headache from a *moño* that pulls the hair too tightly. Doing a dry run will help ensure that your hairdresser is using the right products and techniques for your style on the big day.

Like your makeup artist, your hairdresser will also need to know about conditions at the event that affect the way he or she approaches your hairstyle. Hair behaves differently indoors, outdoors, in the heat of summer in humid Miami, or in the dry, cold air of a Chicago winter.

Beauty for the **Big Day**

SINCE YOU HAVE HAD A TEST RUN FOR both hair and makeup, you will have a good sense of what the batting order should be on the actual day. If, for example, you will use hot rollers in your hair, get them in first and move on to starting the makeup application while the rollers set. As a general rule, unless you hair is very elaborate and complicated, allow two to three hours before the wedding to begin hair and makeup.

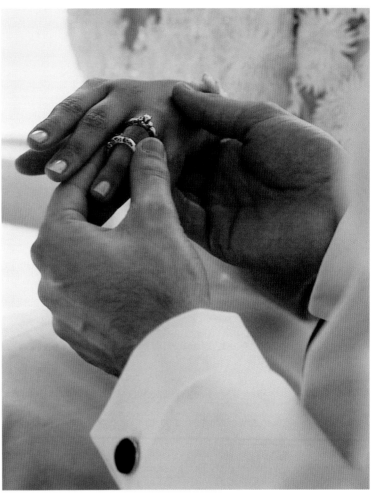

Since all eyes will be on you, keep the beauty details, like your nails, as simple as possible.

You should already have discussed and tried out the makeup palette with your makeup artists and made any adjustments to the look. On the big day, however, life's little surprises—blemishes, bags under the eyes—may make an uninvited visit, so it's best to be prepared. Place some of the following items in a small purse or makeup bag, and have it available when you are ready to start applying your makeup. This kit will also be handy when you are about to take the portraits:

• Redness-reducing eyedrops, to apply to the eyes before makeup application and on any new blemishes to dull redness.

• Oil-blotting papers. Chances are, you may feel quite nervous at various points throughout the day. Nerves can easily cause an extra-oily T-zone—even if you tend to have normal-to-dry skin. Because of this, it is essential to have blotting papers on hand.

- Pressed face powder
- Waterproof mascara
- Eyelash curler—when your eyes get moist with *emoción*, a quick press of the lashes keeps you looking alert and bright instead of *como una histérica*.
- Lipstick
- Many, many tissues

After the makeup artist has applied the base, concealer, and cheek color, and before he or she goes for the rest of the face, request that they apply, with a sponge or a puff, some extra loose powder on your T-zone. As they apply it, they should press the puff onto the face, instead of using the sponge or puff to lightly dust a coating over the entire face. You want the powder to stay in place on the face to provide extra oil-absorbing protection. If you have oily skin, it's a good idea to repeat this extra application once more after the dress is on, the hair is done, and you are almost ready to go. It will give you even more oil-absorption. Once the makeup artist has prepared a good "face" he or she is ready to do the eyes.

You may have a million reasons to do this in a different order, but in general, moving on to hair after eye makeup is applied is a good idea. Have the hairdresser do as much of the hair as possible before putting on the dress. While the hairdresser is probably using heat implements to style, you want to stay cool and fresh, and a wedding dress can sometimes be restrictive and heavy.

After all makeup except the lipstick has been applied, and the hair is almost completely done except for attaching the veil, apply the fragrance. Be mindful of the type of fragrance you are wearing. Perfume, for example, is very strong and should be applied sparingly. Less is more.

Now you are ready to put on the dress and use some tissues. Once you are in the dress, take numerous tissues and tuck one side of each along the neckline of the dress, almost like a bib. Have the makeup artist apply a light coating of bronzing powder, or a powder in a color that will even out any shade differences, to your neck and chest. This is to ensure that when you are being photographed, there won't be a huge difference between the skin on your face and the skin on your chest. Most women do have a color difference, especially if they tend to apply SPF-formula sunscreens to the face to protect skin from damage. (Sunscreen should also be applied to any exposed areas of the skin, but women rarely do this regularly.) Also, when it comes to flash photography, powder absorbs light, which is often what makes women's faces look so freakishly white or gray in some photographs. Applying powder to the face, neck, and chest will even out any discoloration, and the powder will absorb the light from flashbulbs in a uniform manner. The tissues help to protect your dress as you apply the powder.

Finish with the hair, quickly but securely attaching the veil or headpiece, and then do the lipstick. Now take once last long look in the mirror in your final moment as a single woman.

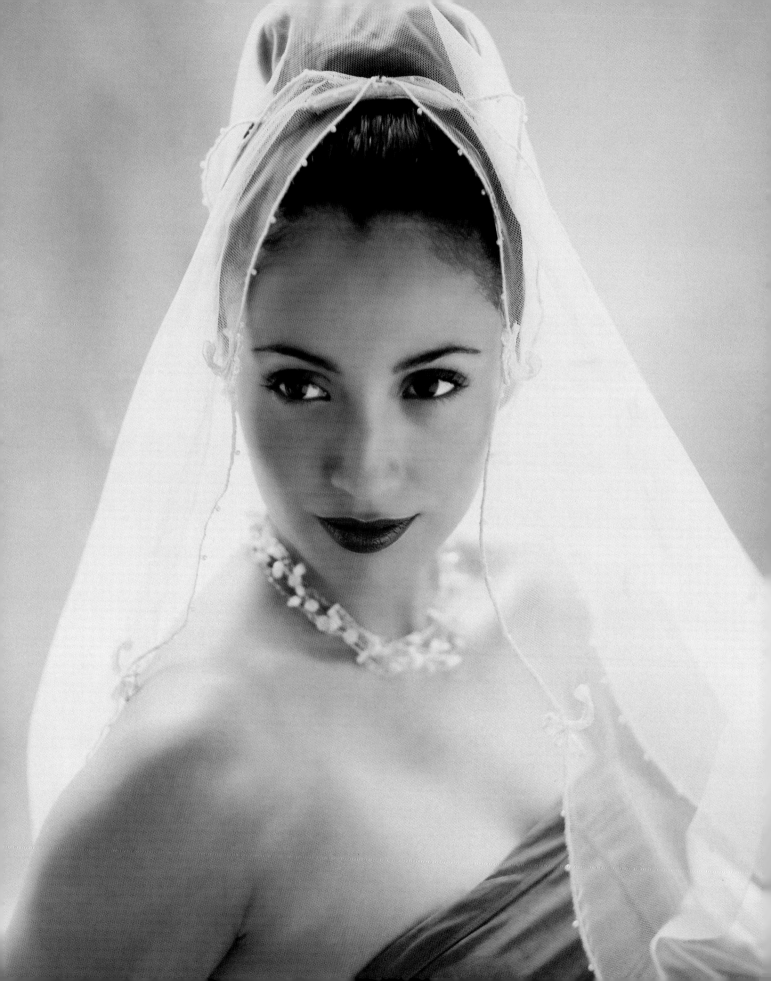

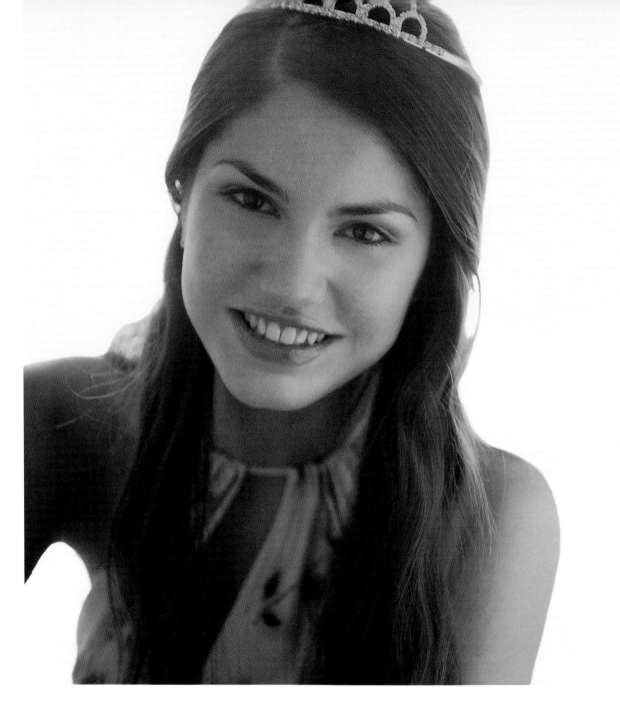

Quinceañeras

IT USED TO BE THAT THE *QUINCEAÑERA* WAS NOT ONLY A FEMALE'S transformation from girl to woman, it was also her introduction into the world of beauty. As many teens already know, girls nowadays tend not to wait for their *corona* before trying and using makeup. By the time the event rolls around the celebrant may be somewhat of an expert who could teach her *mami* a thing or two.

Nonetheless, a *quinceañera* still presents a singular and early lesson about timeless, classical beauty that emphasizes one's own unique features.

With loose hair and shimmery makeup, this *quinceañera* is an example of a more contemporary, modern look that isn't overwhelmed by heavy cosmetics or a too trendy hairstyle.

Makeup, especially when you are young, tends to be an invitation to explore—funky glitter eye pencils, shiny lip gloss, trendy nail polish. After all, this is when you are figuring out the fundamentals of who you are and how you want to express yourself. So it's the time to experiment as much as possible, discovering what looks best and inspires the most confidence.

But a *quinceañera* is a special day. Symbolically, this is the day a girl becomes a woman in the eyes of family and friends. The ideal is to create a beautiful, dignified, and classical passage into adulthood that will be remembered fondly by many, but most important, by the young woman herself.

In some ways, a *quinceañera* is more complicated than a wedding. A wedding is about, or should be about, the creation of a new family through the joining of two adults who are very much in love. Hence it follows that the ceremony, the dress, and every detail about the wedding should, as much as possible, be whatever makes the groom and the bride happy. Of course, a few concessions to the family are to be expected in order to keep people satisfied, but by and large, it is about the couple and what they want. Moreover, in our times, it is not unusual for the couple to carry part if not all of the cost of the wedding.

A *quinceañera* is different. A *quinceañera* is much more about tradition, and much more about family, or, to be more specific, the parents and what they want for their daughter. To put it in even simpler terms, Mom and Dad are most likely footing the entire bill for this *fiesta*, and that drives its dynamics as well as the issues surrounding how the honoree will look. So for the 14-year-old herself, the *quinceañera* becomes an introduction to navigating, in a mature fashion, the negotiations that are a part of every large family function. This is her day; she is the star—and she is generally given a lot of leeway to make all sorts of decisions. This is precisely why every effort should be made to ensure that those decisions are intelligent and well informed. The best overall advice for a young lady planning her *quinceañera*: Think about the big picture, about how you want to experience this day and how you want to remember it years from now, when your daughter is ready for her *quinceañera*.

• **If you have a very clear idea of what you want, take the lead.** Other family members may not like what you have chosen for yourself in terms of makeup and a hairstyle, but unless it misrepresents your age (see tip below) or could be viewed as disrespectful, there is little reason to change dramatically what you are trying to create for yourself.

• **Simple is better.** If there is anything exaggerated about your regular, everyday appearance—from brightly colored hair to huge, rake-like bangs to big, baggy clothes to a preponderance of the color black—let it go for this special day. Appearance is an important thing at any age. When you are a teenager, it really serves to define who you are and what you are becoming. If you use hair and makeup to express that you are creative, introspective, rowdy, or even rebellious, that's up to you. On your *quinceañera*, however, what you are hoping to express is that you are making a proud, smooth, and dignified transition into adulthood.

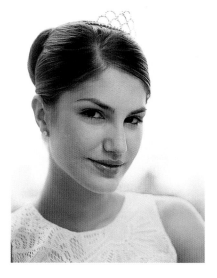

Wearing a proper *moño* and more classic makeup, this *quinceañera* exemplifies a more traditional approach.

It says a lot about someone when she is comfortable enough to be her own person away from her family—in school or among friends—but is savvy enough to understand what the special occasion of the *quinceañera* means in a larger context. It is a chance to express yet another side of the person you are becoming.

• **Make sure that at the end of the hair and makeup session, you still look 15.** This may not be a popular point to make, but it is important nonetheless. The *quinceañera* marks your passage into being a 15-year-old, not a 30-year-old. The idea is not to add years to your look, it is to celebrate the age you are. You may be a 15-year-old who looks 20, even without your makeup and hair done. That's OK—nothing can or should be done to change that. Just stay away from makeup or styling that accentuates this reality. Avoid aging makeup techniques like contouring and hairstyles that are overblown or dated. A good makeup artist and hairstylist will be able to advise you on how to create a look that is fresh and appealing.

• **Stay away from being too trend-oriented.** Brides usually get similar advice. Most stick to it for the same reason you should: It makes for a special-day appearance that is always beautiful. You may be absolutely unwavering on wanting to wear some trend on your *quinceañera*, whether it's bright blond extensions, glitter eye makeup, or a mile-high *moño*. Your *mami* may start telling you you'll regret it two or three years down the line. Listen to what she has to say, and really try to imagine looking at your photos 10, 20 years from now. Do you think you will like what you see? It can also help to look at old photos from *quinceañeras* of various family members—cousins, aunts, even your mother, if she had one. Looking at old photographs is the easy way to learn about the benefits of timeless, classical beauty that always looks elegant. Also, compare an old photograph of Rita Hayworth to an old photograph of Raquel Welch from the '70s. Both look beautiful, of course, but Rita represents an image of ageless grace and beauty that is not dated or trend-oriented.

Stick to makeup color palettes that suit the color scheme of the event. As with brides, it is best to already have picked out the hairstyle and tiara before approaching a makeup artist and hairdresser. That way, they will be able to make the best recommendations given your coloring and the colors you will be wearing. Neutral makeup that is not excessively shiny will photograph well, so your look stays good for years to come.

• **Use the whole experience as a learning opportunity.** If you don't have a superclear idea of what you want, consider your mother's advice on what to do, which dress to select, and what makeup and hairstyle to wear for the big day. Use this as a bonding experience between the two of you, and be thankful that she is sharing her wisdom and experience. (Again, she probably will, anyway.)

One approach may be to look through magazines and pictures of famous Latinas to garner makeup and hair ideas. Another is to visit various salons and to schedule consultations with a few makeup and hair people before both of you settle on what you will do.

• **Take care that any insecurities you may have about your appearance are not magnified by this celebration.** Let's face it: When you are turning 15, you may feel less than comfortable with a lot of things about your appearance. Braces, acne, a body that is still taking shape—all these things are completely normal but can be a source of great anxiety when you are to be presented at a celebration where all eyes are on you. What is commonly forgotten about *quinceañeras* is that they should be fun, not anxiety-ridden. If you have certain issues you are dealing with, the best thing to do—in life in general, as well as for your *quinceañera*—is to do what you can about the things you can control and simply not allow yourself to worry about the things you can't. If skin is the issue, take this opportunity either to go to a dermatologist to have your skin treated, or to initiate a skin-care regimen that you will stick to. Next, learn from a local makeup artist how to cover up blemishes like a pro. These tactics are proactive decisions that will benefit you for the rest of your life. Do you have braces? Your orthodontist probably won't be arranging your tooth-straightening schedule around your *quinceañera* plans, so this issue definitely falls into the "don't worry about it" category. A good makeup artist and hairstylist will work with the braces by making your hair and eyes the focal point, and that *corona* will definitely keep people's eyes away from your teeth.

At the end of these special days, after the *brindis* have been made and the *mariachis* have made everyone cry, your family and community will have welcomed another 15-year-old young lady into its ranks.

Makeup for photography

KNOWING WHAT TYPE OF PHOTOGRAPHS WILL be taken also helps you select the best makeup choices. Are you having an outdoor wedding? A *quinceañera* with a party under the stars? Then adjust your makeup accordingly.

Flash photography

Flash photography can affect the way color shows up on film. White looks whiter; reds and pinks can get washed out. Some women make the mistake of overcompensating by applying too much blush. Lipstick will bring color to your face, and while you may turn up the notch slightly on the amount of blush you wear, be careful to not overdo it.

Outdoor/natural lighting

Natural lighting, while the truest, is also the most brutal for showing flaws. This is why most makeup artists recommend that women stay away from shimmery colors, which can make you look greasy or, if it falls into the fine lines around the eyes, emphasize crow's feet. More than anything, natural lighting will reveal any uneven coloring on the face; blotchiness or redness in certain areas must be carefully blended out.

Apply powder to the chest to avoid having the face look powdery or fake, since, as we mentioned before, powder absorbs light from the photographer's flash.

Positioning your face

For at least a few of the portraits, you may want to get a sense of what your "best angle" is—most women already do know what it is, whether they are aware of it or not. Look through old photographs of yourself and try to determine which angles are most flattering. One interesting point: Although photographers rarely do so at formal weddings, having your picture taken from an angle where the camera is higher than your face, forcing it to become slightly upturned, is a very flattering angle for most people. It elongates and slims down the face.

Makeup touch-up

You might want to consider having the makeup artist do a fast touch-up for the photo session. Be a thoughtful bride and give all of your bridal party the chance to touch up (quickly) before the session starts. If having a makeup artist there is not an option, use the emergency kit we describe on pages 173–74.

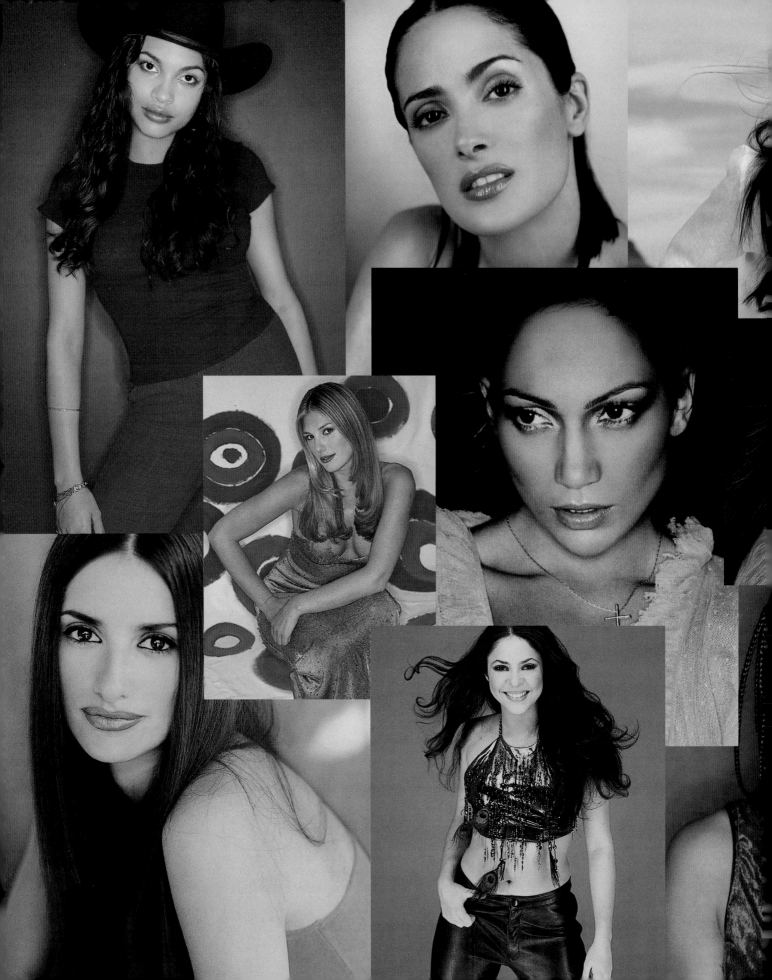

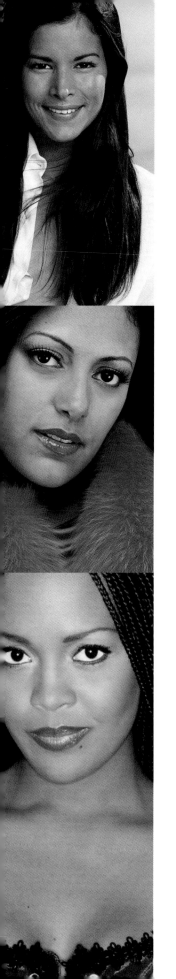

Celebrity *Secretos*

FROM BARELY-THERE MAKEUP TO FAKE EYELASHES, FROM simple hairstyles to hair with extensions, these Latina celebrities teach us how to experiment with our looks and reinvent ourselves with the makeup and hair we choose—or dare—to wear. These women are breaking barriers, setting records, and making the rest of the world stand up and pay attention. Their makeup artists and hairstylists provide the tips and the how-to steps, but these stars provide their own attitude and boldness. Some of the celebrities here have cultivated their singular look. Others break every beauty rule in the book (even this book) and show us how we can do it too.

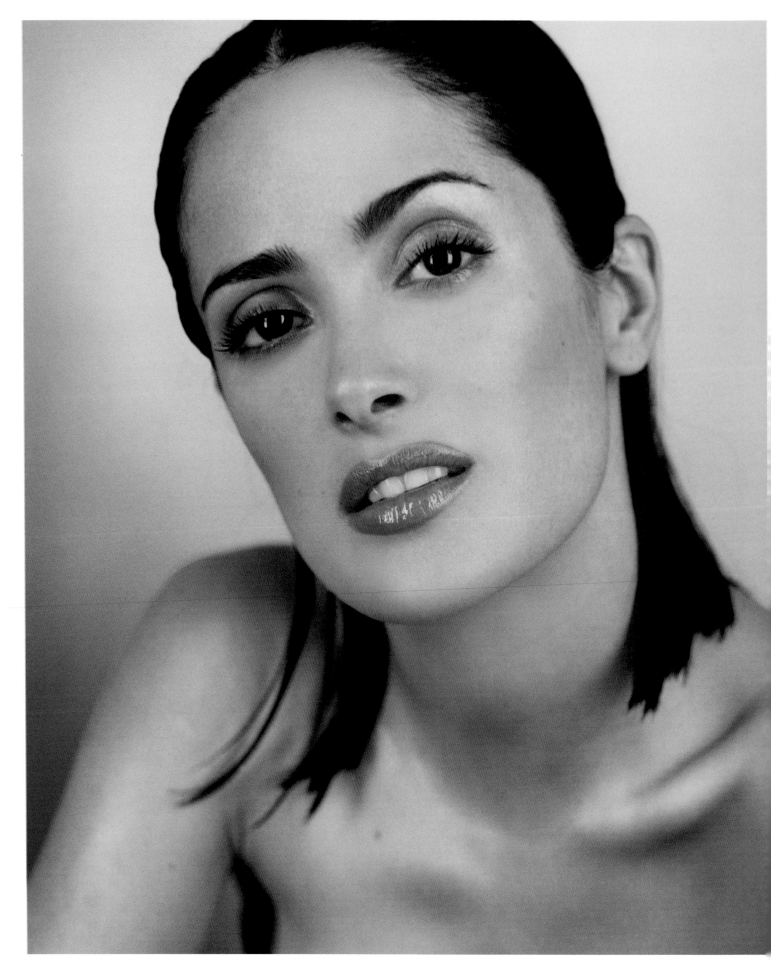

SalmaHayek

SALMA IS WEARING THE *DIEZ MINUTITOS* EYE USING A PALETTE OF SHIMMERY neutrals to accentuate her eye shape. The rest of the face is kept sheer and simple.

Technique

Face:

✔ Apply foundation and concealer to even out skin tone and camouflage any blemishes. Blend well with foundation sponge. Skip the powder—unless you have oily skin—since the face should be left with a slightly dewy, fresh texture.

✔ Use a dark contour powder lightly mixed with blush to give definition to the hollows of the cheeks while lending a slight color to the face. Since you are not applying face powder, go easy on the contour and blush, using the brush to blend well.

Eyes:

✔ Prepare the eye area with concealer. (A brightening formula will work best with this look.)

✔ Apply a neutral pink or pearl eye shadow with a slight sheen in the formula over the entire eyelid area, including the brow bone, using the all-over eye-shadow brush.

✔ Use the platinum, silver, or slightly violet frosty shadow as contour. Beginning at the outer edge of the eye, apply the color along the crease of the brow bone, blending well with the contour brush.

✔ Apply a line of the light-gray shimmery eye shadow along the outer two-thirds of the upper and lower lash line using the powder eyeliner brush. Blend up and outward to create a shiny, slightly smoky effect.

✔ Use the shimmery white highlighter shadow on the outer two-thirds of the brow bone, directly under the brow. Blend well with all-over eye-shadow brush.

✔ Curl lashes and finish eyes with one to two coats of black mascara.

Makeup tools

- **foundation**
- **foundation sponge**
- **concealer**
- **dark contour powder**
- **contour powder brush**
- **blush**
- **blush brush**
- **brightening-formula eye concealer**
- **neutral pink or pearl eye shadow**
- **all-over eye-shadow brush**
- **platinum, silver, or slightly violet, frosty contour shadow**
- **contour eye-shadow brush**
- **light-gray iridescent eye shadow**
- **powder eyeliner brush**
- **shimmery white highlighter shadow**
- **eyelash curler**
- **black mascara**
- **brow gel**
- **neutral, skin-tone lip liner**
- **clear or pink gloss**

Hair tools

- **styling cream**
- **styling gel**
- **a large, flat, oval brush**
- **small, flat bobby pins**

✔ Brows should be kept groomed and clean, but not overly plucked or penciled in. Inner eyebrow hairs are combed up and left up. Seal the brow hairs with a light coating of brow gel.

Lips:

✔ With a neutral brownish-pink lip liner, line the lips using gentle, feathered strokes. Do not draw a thick line, since liner is only being used in this case to bring out definition and to shape the lips.

✔ Select a clear or a pink gloss for the lips to give shine. Note that the lips' texture shows through the gloss; don't load the lips with a thick application or the effect will be heavy-handed.

Hair:

✔ Begin with straight hair. (If you don't have it naturally, create it with the blow-dry technique described on p. 82.) Apply generous amounts of a mixture of styling cream and gel, starting from the hairline and working backward toward the ends. (Styling cream helps smooth the hair while minimizing the sticky hold of the gel.) If your hair is naturally straight, you can also use water to dampen the hair. Avoid this if your hair is naturally curly, however, since the water will cause the hair to frizz.

✔ Use the flat, oval brush to smooth hair back, keeping it close to the head.

✔ Tuck the sides behind the ears and use small, flat bobby pins to secure in place. If you have wavy or curly hair, secure the back of the hair with pins as well to prevent poufing as the product dries in the hair.

Daisy**Fuentes**

CLASSICAL MAKEUP WITH SMOOTH LOCKS
create a sleek, sophisticated look.

Technique

Face:

✔ Begin by tweezing any excess hair from eyebrows to create a classic, smooth shape.

✔ Using the foundation brush, apply concealer to areas requiring coverage, targeting spots like the edges of the nose where redness occurs.

✔ Follow with an application of foundation, applying dots of foundation down the sides of the face to ensure even distribution, then blend with the brush.

✔ To blend foundation at the neck line, apply dots on the chin and blend downward using a makeup sponge.

✔ Apply rose-colored blush to the cheeks.

✔ Using a powder brush, apply a coat of translucent powder over the entire face, including the eyelids. This sets the foundation, concealer, and blush.

Eyes:

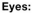

✔ Create contours in the eye area to enhance the shape. Start by applying a brown eye shadow with a contour brush to the outer two-thirds of the eye along the crease.

✔ Using eyeliner brush and with the same brown eye shadow placed in the crease, apply eye shadow along the top lash line. The end result is a V-shape that meets at the corner of the eye. Blend lines very well.

✔ For extra-smoky eyes, apply black eyeliner over the brown shadow, smudging the eyeliner as you go. Apply a light dusting of translucent powder over the eye to set color.

✔ Use eyelash curler on lashes, followed by an application of mascara.

Lips:

✔ Line the lips with a nude-colored lip pencil.

✔ Fill in lips with a matching lip color. There should be no harsh line between lip liner and color.

✔ Apply a coat of clear lip gloss over the entire mouth to impart a high shine.

Hair:

✔ Begin with straight hair, natural or created with our blow-drying techniques.

✔ Divide hair into two-to-three-inch sections. Apply a small amount of a moisturizing hairdressing cream to one section, concentrating on the ends.

✔ Use the round, flat brush to ensure that the product has been well distributed, on the ends in particular, and that the hair is smooth and tangle-free.

✔ Hold section taut, and using the straightening iron beginning near the roots place the prepared section of hair between the clamps. Bring the iron down in a slow, fluid movement to avoid creasing the hair.

✔ Repeat procedure on all the sections of hair until finished.

Makeup tools

- **synthetic bristled foundation brush (for foundation and concealer)**
- **concealer**
- **foundation**
- **foundation sponge**
- **rose blush**
- **blush brush**
- **translucent loose powder**
- **contour eye-shadow brush**
- **brown eye shadow**
- **powder eyeliner brush**
- **black eyeliner**
- **eyelash curler**
- **mascara**
- **nude lip pencil**
- **nude lip color**
- **clear lip gloss**

Hair tools

- **hairdressing cream**
- **flat oval brush**
- **straightening iron**

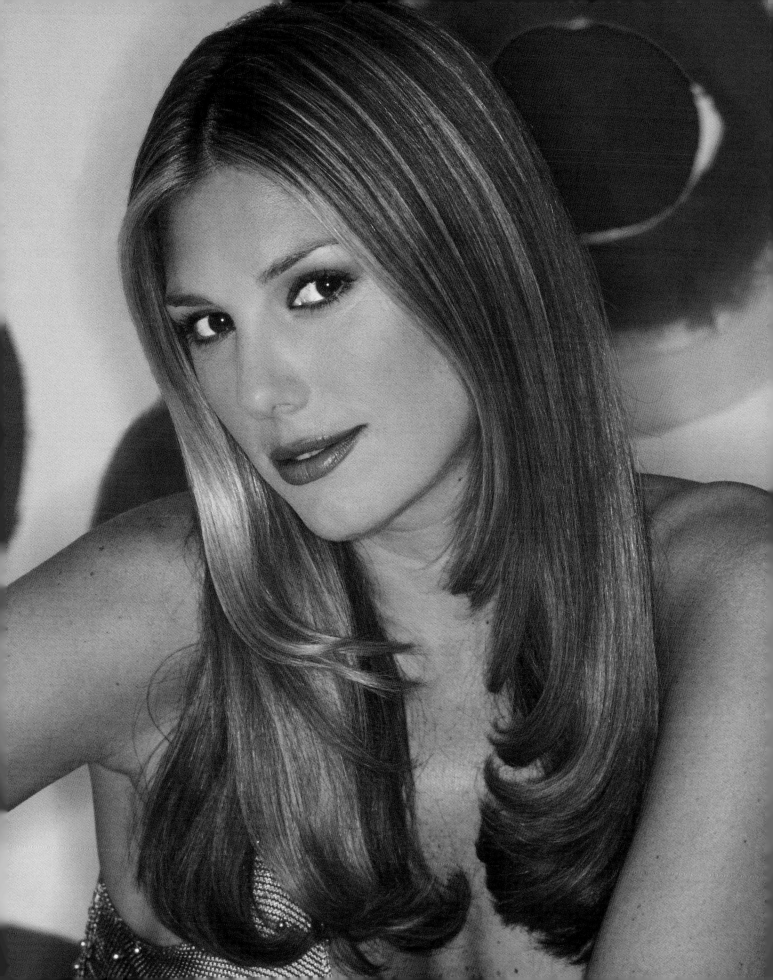

MagaliCaicedo

COLOR IS THE KEY TO RECREATING MAGALI'S LOOK. PINKS AND BLUES keep things sweet, while contouring helps bring out beautiful bone structure.

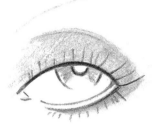

Technique

Face:

✔ Apply concealer to areas that need extra coverage, blending well.

✔ Several different-colored foundations were used on Magali. To keep things simple, use a foundation to even out skin tone and dark contour powder to shape the face.

✔ Use contour brush to apply contour powder in the hollows of the cheeks.

✔ Apply a bit of rose-tinged blush to the cheeks to give slight color.

✔ Blend contour and blush with a powder puff, leaving no clear demarcation lines. The goal is to bring out the existing bone structure.

Eyes:

✔ Apply a sheer, shimmery eye shadow all over the eyelid and on the inner corner of the eye, including the bottom inner corner.

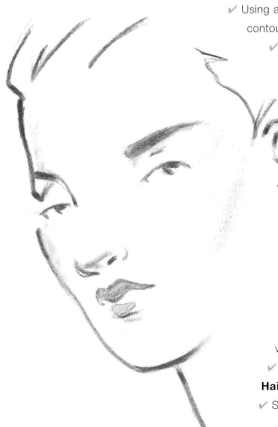

✔ Using a light-blue eye shadow, apply color to the crease of the eyelid with a contour brush.

✔ Apply black cake eyeliner along the top lash line with liquid eyeliner brush.

✔ Use a soft-brown eyeliner to line the bottom lash line.

✔ Using eyebrow brush, apply a medium-brown eyebrow powder to thicken thin brows and create a more prominent frame for the eye. Stay true to the brow shape, since the goal is to accentuate the brow, not to create a whole new one.

✔ Curl lashes and follow with a coat of mascara.

Lips:

✔ Prepare the lips with foundation to even out lips with variations of pigment, like Magali's. Apply a light dusting of powder over the foundation to set the lips.

✔ Follow with the lip liner. Use a light hand to give definition to the lip shape.

✔ Apply the lighter lip color. This accentuates the lip's shape. Blend well, since there should be no harsh line between the lip liner and color.

✔ Follow with an application of pink gloss.

Hair:

✔ Spray the braids with sheen to give them shine.

Makeup tools

- **concealer**
- **foundation**
- **foundation sponge**
- **contour powder**
- **contour brush**
- **rose-toned blush**
- **powder puff**
- **sheer, shimmery eye shadow**
- **light blue eye shadow**
- **liqiud eyeliner brush**
- **black cake eyeliner**
- **brown eyeliner**
- **medium-brown eyebrow powder**
- **dark lip liner**
- **lighter, salmon-colored lipstick**
- **frosty pink gloss**

Hair tools

- **braid sheen oil**
- **elastic ponytail holder**

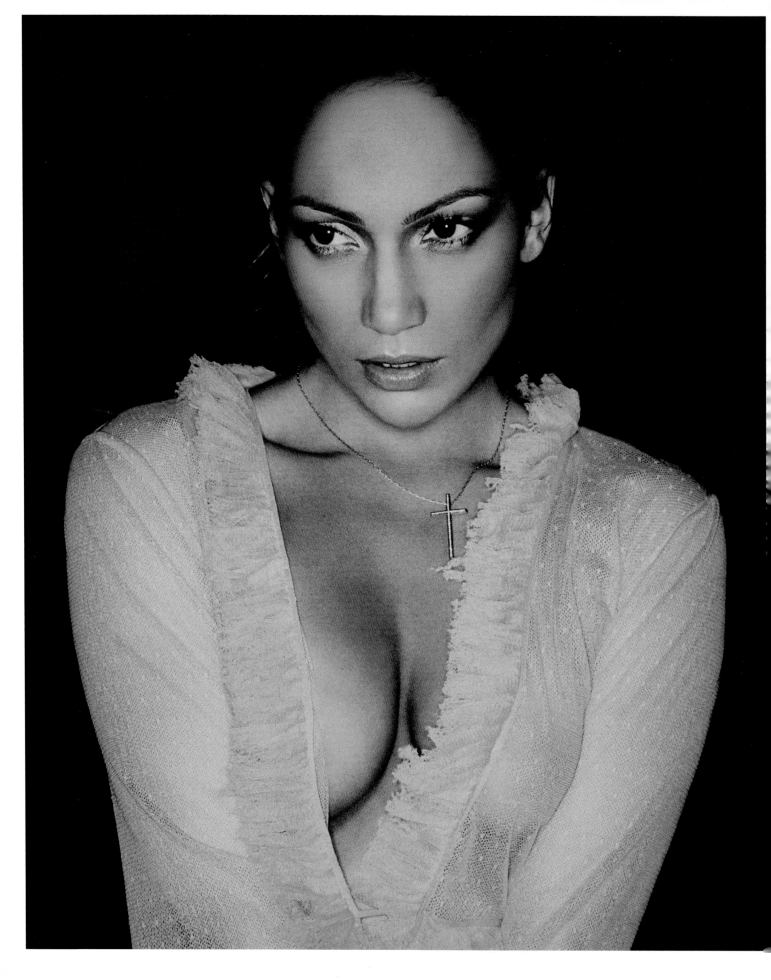

Jennifer**Lopez**

AN EDGIER, MODERN LOOK BRINGS THE EYES INTO FOCUS. SIMPLE, SWEPT-back hair prevents it from looking overdone.

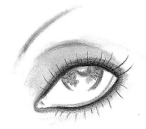

Technique

Face:

✔ Apply foundation to the face, using fingers to help the color "melt" into the skin, leaving a flawless finish.

✔ Use reflective concealer sparingly around the eyes.

✔ Use foundation sponge to "buff" the makeup, blending the colors.

✔ Apply cream blush with fingers, starting at the apples of the cheeks and blending back into the hollows to define bone structure.

✔ Skip powder, since skin should impart a sheer, polished glow.

Eyes:

✔ Tweeze brows into a strong shape.

✔ With fingertips, apply charcoal cream eye shadow from the center of the eyelid up to the crease.

✔ Apply gray metallic liquid eye shadow along the upper and lower lash lines, including the inner eye area. Make the line of eye shadow rather thick using the contour eye-shadow brush. It will be blended in the next step with the black eyeliner.

✔ Using black eyeliner pencil, draw a thin line along the top lash line and lightly along the lower lash line. Smudge the line gently to create a smoky effect.

✔ Curl natural lashes.

✔ Using tweezers, apply individual fake eyelashes along the top lash line. Apply eyelash adhesive to the end of each bunch, and wait a count of 30 seconds before anchoring the fake lash along the natural lash line. Use a total of about ten bunches per eye.

✔ Use brown eyebrow pencil to fill in and accentuate brow shape.

✔ With eyebrow brush, brush the brows into place, blending the color of the eyebrow pencil into the brow.

✔ Seal brow color and shape with eyebrow gel.

Lips:

✔ Line lips with a liner that matches your natural lip color. This will give definition without adding excess color.

✔ Smooth over a generous amount of the silver-beige lip gloss.

Hair:

✔ Begin with straight hair, and finish ends with silicon drops to ensure that hair stays smooth.

✔ Using the oval, flat brush, smooth all the hair back and away from the face. Make sure no part is left in the hair.

✔ Pull into a ponytail at the back of the head. Secure with the elastic band.

✔ Apply pomade to the sides and top to keep hair smooth and shiny. Rub a dab of pomade between the palms, then carefully smooth them over the pulled-back hair.

✔ Use fingers to gently style the tiny, fine "baby" hairs along the hairline. Bring them forward to frame the face, giving the style a youthful quality.

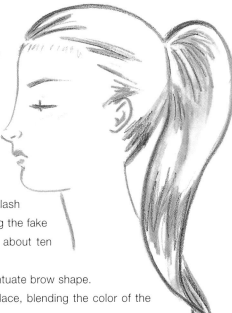

Makeup tools

- **liquid foundation**
- **brightening concealer**
- **foundation sponge**
- **brownish-pink cream blush**
- **charcoal cream eye shadow**
- **gray metallic liquid eye shadow**
- **contour eye-shadow brush**
- **individual false eyelashes**
- **tweezers**
- **eyelash adhesive**
- **eyelash curler**
- **mascara**
- **brown eyebrow pencil**
- **eye brow brush**
- **eyebrow gel**
- **nude lip liner**
- **silver-beige lip gloss**

Hair tools

- **oval, flat brush**
- **pomade with gold flecks**
- **silicone hair serum**
- **elastic ponytail holder**

RosarioDawson

ROSARIO'S MAKEUP IS GLOWING AND FRESH. HAIR IS KEPT LOOSE, TOUSLED, AND TEXTURED TO ACCENT the youthful, relaxed appeal.

Technique

Face:

✔ Apply sheer foundation and concealer to even out skin tone. As with Salma's look (page 183), skip the powder unless you have oily skin, since the face should be left with a slightly dewy, fresh texture.

✔ Use a pink blush on the apples of the cheeks to give a hint of color. Blend well with brush.

Eyes:

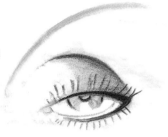

✔ Prepare the eye area with concealer; use a brightening formula and apply sparingly.

✔ Apply a pink eye shadow with a slight sheen in the formula across the entire eyelid area, including the brow bone, using the all-over eye-shadow brush. Extend up to the brow, since this color will serve as your highlighter on the brow bone.

✔ Use the contour brush to apply the shimmery white shadow to the inner corners of the eye. The shadow should extend slightly to the top and bottom inner rims.

✔ Beginning at the outer edge of the eye, apply shimmery peach shadow along the crease of the brow bone as your contour color, blending well with the contour brush.

✔ Use the powder eyeliner brush to apply a line of dark-brown eye shadow along the outer two-thirds of the upper and lower lash lines. Apply this only to give definition to the outer part of the eye. Don't be too heavy-handed with the eye shadow; the end effect is a pair of glowing, sexy eyes.

✔ Curl lashes and finish eyes with one coat of black mascara.

✔ Brows should be kept natural yet groomed. Tweeze any stray hairs and, if necessary, keep the hairs in place with a light coating of brow gel.

Makeup Tools

- **sheer foundation**
- **foundation sponge**
- **concealer**
- **pink blush**
- **blush brush**
- **brightening formula eye concealer**
- **pink eye shadow**
- **shimmery white eye shadow**
- **an all-over eye-shadow brush**
- **peach contour eye shadow**
- **contour eye-shadow brush**
- **dark-brown eye shadow**
- **powder eyeliner brush**
- **eyelash curler**
- **black mascara**
- **brow gel**
- **neutral, skin-tone lip liner**
- **pink gloss**

Hair Tools

- **conditioning hairdressing cream**
- **wide-tooth comb**
- **blow-dryer**
- **silicon hair serum**

Lips:

✔ With a neutral pink-tone lip liner, line the lips using gentle, feathered strokes.

✔ Apply a generous coating of shimmery pink gloss on the lips.

Hair:

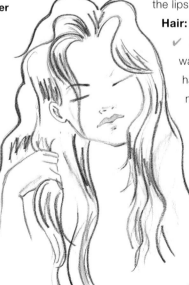

✔ Begin with slightly damp hair, either freshly washed or misted with a water sprayer. Rosario's hair is naturally wavy, and these styling techniques build on her natural texture.

✔ Apply conditioning cream to the hair. Use the wide-tooth comb to ensure that the product is evenly distributed.

✔ Use blow-dryer and style with fingers as you dry to loosen waves and create tousled, lanky locks.

✔ Once hair is dry, use silicon hair serum to prevent frizzies. Place a few drops on the palms, then rub them together and run them over the hair, focusing on the ends.

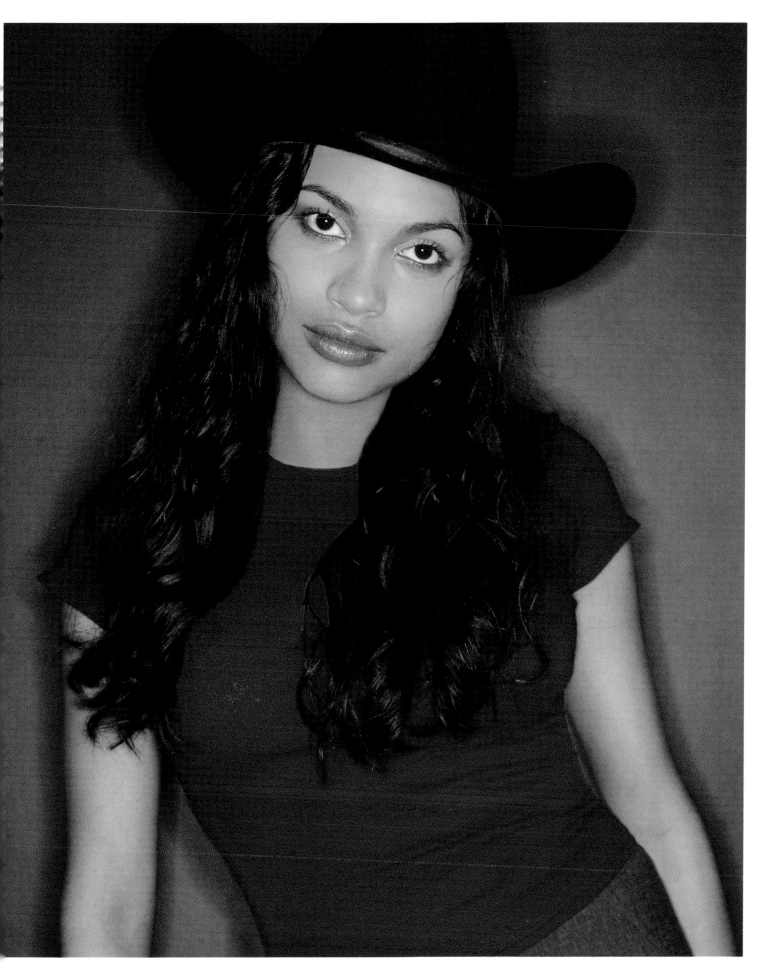

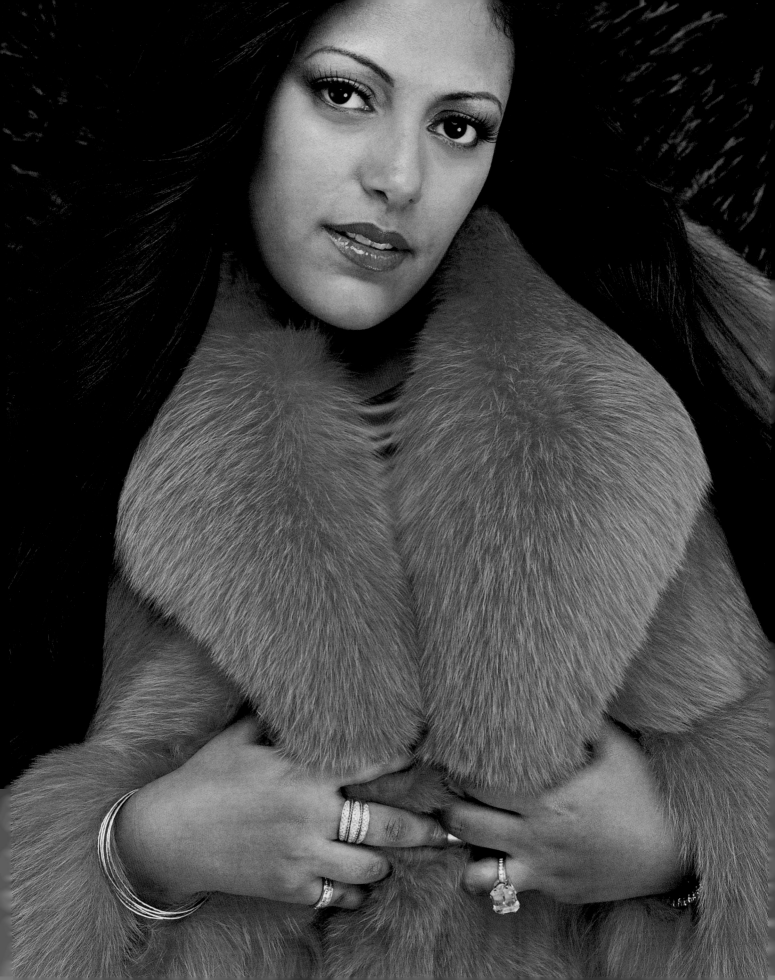

La India

WITH A PAIR OF DRAMATIC LASHES, THE REST OF THE makeup is simple. Smooth, soft hair completes the look.

Technique

Face:

✔ Apply liquid foundation to even out skin tone. Use foundation brush to blend evenly.

✔ Use concealer around the eye, again blending with foundation brush. Mix concealer with foundation if necessary to ensure evenness of tone.

✔ Use cream blush to add a slight color to the cheeks. Blend with fingers.

✔ Apply loose powder with puff to lightly set makeup. The skin should look luminous, not matte, so go easy on the powder.

Eyes:

✔ Use all-over eye shadow brush to apply brown eye shadow to entire lid.

✔ With a powder eyeliner brush, apply the same brown eye shadow to lightly rim the lower lash line.

✔ Follow with the black eyeliner pencil on the top and bottom lash line, going over the brown eye shadow to create a slightly more dramatic (but not heavy-handed) look. Draw a very thin line along the bottom lashes and a thicker one along the top lashes.

✔ With finger, blend the top line for a smoky effect.

✔ Apply a line of eyelash adhesive to the strip of false lashes. Wait a count of 30 seconds before placing the strip along the top lash line.

✔ To give more shape to thin brows, use the eyebrow pencil to fill in and accentuate the natural arch of the brow.

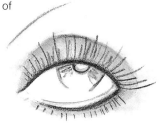

Lips:

✔ Skip the lip pencil. Instead, use the pink-beige lipstick to give a hint of color.

✔ Follow with a generous application of high-shine clear lip gloss.

Makeup tools

- **liquid foundation**
- **foundation brush**
- **concealer**
- **loose face powder**
- **powder puff**
- **brownish-pink blush**
- **charcoal-brown eye shadow**
- **all-over eye-shadow brush**
- **eyeliner brush**
- **black eyeliner pencil**
- **mascara**
- **false eyelashes**
- **eyelash adhesive**
- **brown eyebrow pencil**
- **pink-beige lipstick**
- **clear lip gloss**

Hair tools

- **volumizing spray**
- **large-barrel curling iron**
- **large Velcro rollers**
- **large oval brush**
- **silicon hair serum**

Hair:

✔ Apply volumizing spray to hair, concentrating on the roots for lift.

✔ Using a large-barrel curling iron, curl the hair in sections to smooth and lift.

✔ After each section is curled, wrap it in a large Velcro roller. The rollers give shape and body to the hair while still keeping it smooth.

✔ Remove rollers after the hair has cooled and set.

✔ Brush out the hair with a large oval brush.

✔ Pour a few drops of hair serum into the hands. Apply the serum by rubbing palms together and then lightly over the surface of the hair. Concentrate on the ends to make them smooth and eliminate flyaway hairs.

Penélope**Cruz**

Makeup tools

- **liquid foundation**
- **foundation sponge**
- **translucent powder**
- **loose powder brush**
- **rose-colored powder blush**
- **blush brush**
- **cream- or gold-tinted
  eye shadow**
- **all-over eye-shadow brush**
- **dark brown eye shadow**
- **powder eye-shadow brush**
- **black eyeliner pencil**
- **black mascara**
- **pinkish brown lip liner**
- **pink lip gloss**

Hair tools

- **straightening balm**
- **hair dryer with straightening
  nozzle**
- **large round brush**
- **flat iron**
- **silicon drops**
- **round flat brush**

SMOOTH, SLEEK HAIR FRAMES BLACK eyeliner–rimmed eyes and simple lips.

Technique

Face:

✔ Apply liquid foundation to give medium coverage to the skin, evening out discolorations. Blend with sponge.

✔ Set makeup and give a matte finish to the face with an application of translucent powder. Use the loose powder blush to apply the translucent powder evenly over the face.

✔ Apply a light dusting of rose-colored blush to the cheeks. This gives the skin a hint of color, since the lips are very light.

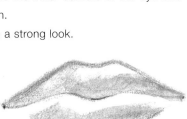

Eyes:

✔ Prepare the eyes with a light application of concealer under the eyes and on the lids. Since the lids will only have a light color on them, the skin tone needs to be evened out.

✔ Apply the cream- or gold-tinted eye shadow with the all-over eye-shadow brush. The eye shadow should cover the entire lid, but especially the brow bone, as it works as a highlighter.

✔ Use the powder eyeliner brush to apply a line of dark brown eye shadow along the top lash line. Be sure to apply the shadow close to the lash line, creating a smokiness emphasized by thin lines.

✔ With the black eyeliner pencil, line the entire lower inner rim of the eye. Then line the inner corners of the eye and finish with a light line along the top lash line. Again, the lines should be kept very thin.

✔ Apply a light coat of mascara. Apply sparingly, since the black eyeliner gives such a strong look.

Lips:

✔ Finish the face with lips that are defined but not overpowering.

✔ Use the pinkish-brown neutral liner to line the lips, giving them a nice shape and strong edge. Fill in lips with liner to keep the color long-lasting and to cut down on the shine from the gloss.

✔ Follow with an application of gloss over the lips. Since the look here is not shiny and hard, use lip gloss that gives more color than shine, and apply just enough so that the lips are left looking moist but not greasy.

Hair:

✔ Begin with straight hair. (Penelope's was blow-dried straight, using a hairdryer with a straightening nozzle, a large round brush, and a straightening balm to relax the waves.)

✔ Divide hair into two-to-three-inch sections. Add silicon drops to keep it from frizzing.

✔ Use the round flat brush to ensure product has been well distributed, on the ends in particular, and to make sure hair is smooth and tangle-free.

✔ Hold section taught, and, using the straightening iron beginning near the roots, place the section of hair between the clamps. Bring the iron down the section of hair in a slow, fluid movement to avoid creasing the hair.

✔ Style hair by parting in the middle and brushing the hair evenly for a very sleek, modern look.

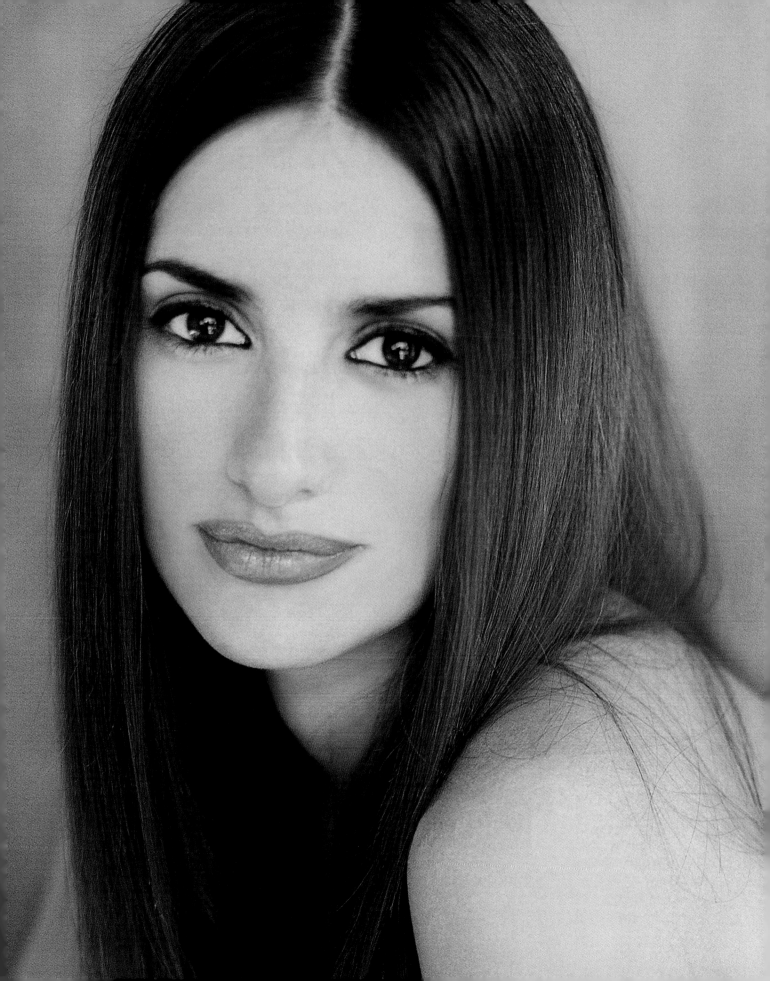

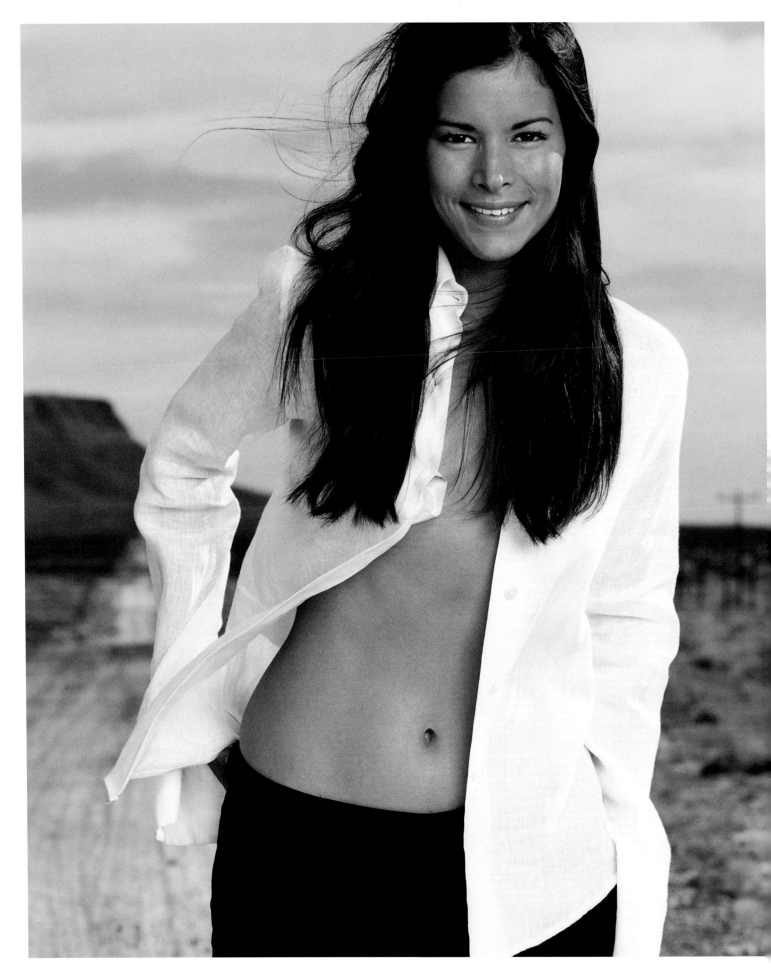

Patricia**Velasquez**

MAKEUP FOR THIS LOOK IS MINIMAL, REQUIRING ALMOST FLAWLESS SKIN. The hair, on the other hand, can get tricky, although the intended result looks effortless and "natural."

Technique

Face:

✔ Apply a light coat of foundation all over the face to cover any unevenness in skin tone. Blend well with fingers.

✔ Since this is a fresh, simple look, skip the blush.

Eyes:

✔ Apply shimmery golden shadow on lids using all-over shadow brush.

Lips:

✔ Lip liner would appear too harsh compared with the rest of the face. Simply use the lip brush to apply the shimmery, soft pink–colored gloss for a wash of color.

Hair:

✔ Begin with straight hair (natural or blow-dried).

✔ Separate and section off the top layer of hair around the crown. Secure it with a hair clip to keep it out of the way as you apply the extensions.

✔ Select extensions in a color and texture that matches your own. The extensions are meant to add volume and thickness in this case, not texture or highlights.

✔ Using extensions glue, adhere rows of human hair extensions starting at the back of the head.

✔ After each row has been anchored to the scalp, blend the extension with the natural hair by bringing down a top layer and brushing the natural and fake hair together.

✔ Repeat procedure, placing the next row of hair in another area at the back or sides of the head. Four sections of Patricia's hair had extensions glued on.

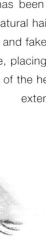

✔ After the hair has been attached and brushed, and the hair from the top of the hair let down, cut the extensions so that they match the length of the natural hair. Cutting with the extensions in also lets the real and fake hair blend a bit better.

Makeup tools

- **foundation**
- **golden shimmery eye shadow**
- **all-over eye-shadow brush**
- **lip brush**
- **pink shimmery lip gloss**

Hair tools

- **volumizing spray**
- **human hair extentions**
- **extensions glue**
- **hair clip**
- **brush**
- **comb**

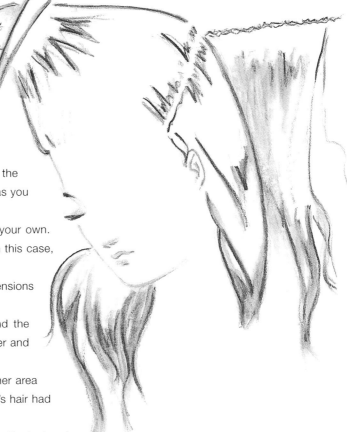

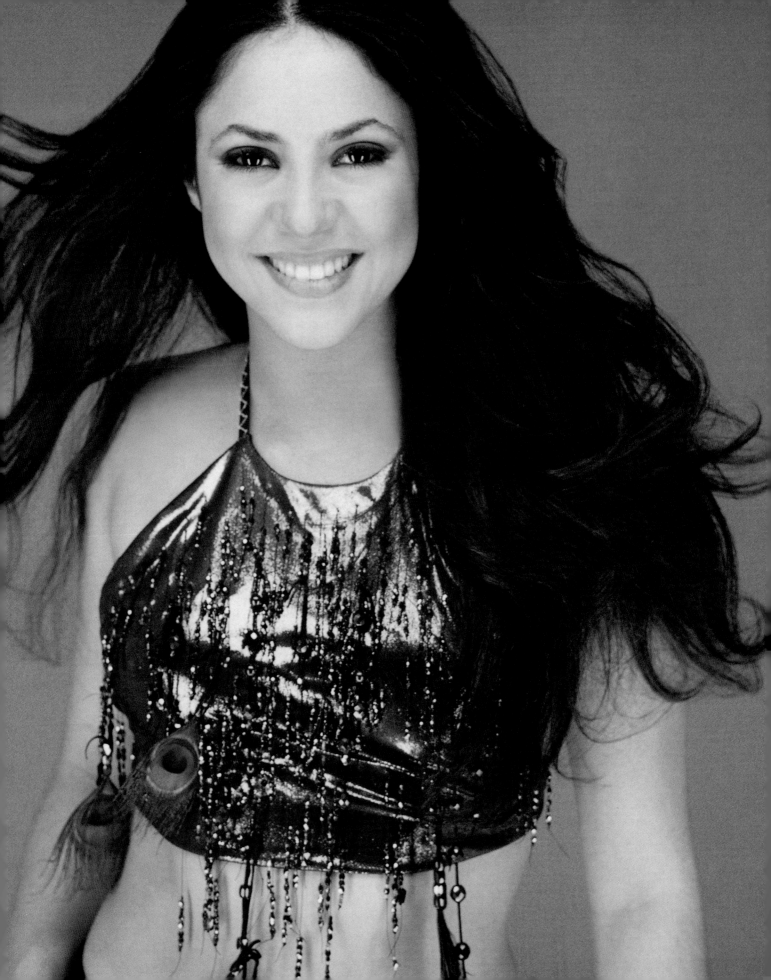

Shakira

BREAKING BEAUTY RULES GALORE AND CREATING A BOHEMIAN LOOK THAT is still feminine, Shakira is an example of highly individual beauty style.

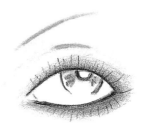

Technique

Face:

✔ Apply concealer to areas that need extra coverage. Go lightly around the eye area, since a fair amount of makeup will be applied later.

✔ Using the foundation sponge to blend, smooth a thin layer of foundation over the face.

✔ Shakira breaks many beauty rules and manages to make them work for her. The first: Her pink-toned blush is applied not to the apples of the cheeks, but underneath. This looks good on her because the color is light enough to add a youthful rosiness to her face. Use this technique, but remember to go very lightly with the blush and blend well.

✔ Finish the face with a light dusting of loose powder to match your skin tone. Be sure to apply a generous amount under the eye area.

Eyes:

✔ Using the powder eyeliner brush, apply purple eye shadow around the entire eye, staying close to the lash line. Think of it as doing a smoky eye, except you are using purple instead of the traditional gray or dark brown. Using a contour brush, apply more purple eyeshadow over the ball of the eyelid.

✔ The second rule she breaks: While most women don't apply eyeliner to the inner rim of the lower lids because it makes the eyes look smaller, Shakira does it anyway and manages to pull it off. Using a black eyeliner pencil, lightly line the inner rim of the lower lash line.

✔ Use the black eyeliner on the top lash line as well, making a slightly thicker, more smudged line.

✔ Blend the black eyeliner and the purple eye shadow along the top lash line using the eyeliner brush.

✔ Curl the lashes and apply mascara.

✔ Leave brows as natural as possible, doing only minimal grooming.

Lips:

✔ Use a pink-tone lip liner to define the lip line.

✔ Follow with a light application of creamy pink lipstick. The lips are kept soft.

Hair:

✔ Here, Shakira breaks a third rule. At a petite 5'2", she wears her hair far below the "bra line length" most stylists (and we in this book) recommend. How does she pull it off yet again? She makes the length of her hair part of her bohemian-chic look.

✔ This style would work well with virtually any hair texture. It lends itself to curly hair, wavy hair, and straight—as long as it is your natural hair texture. If you want to replicate the look exactly, however, begin with straight or wavy hair. Use a large-barreled curling iron to create a bend and a slight curve—but not curl—at the ends.

✔ Don't curl all the ends; leave some pieces alone. (Shakira has some wave to her hair naturally.)

✔ To eliminate frizz but keep hair flexible, use a hair serum. Pour a drop of the serum into the hands. Rub together and apply it by rubbing the palms lightly over the surface of the hair, especially on the ends.

✔ Using the hands, lightly scrunch the loose ends. This is to give it a loose feel with lots of movement.

✔ Let the hair fall naturally, without a strongly defined part.

Makeup tools

- concealer
- foundation
- foundation sponge
- pink-toned blush
- blush brush
- loose powder
- purple eye shadow
- black eyeliner
- powder eyeliner brush
- contour brush
- pink-tone lip liner
- creamy or sheer pink lipstick

Hair tools

- large-barreled curling iron
- hair serum

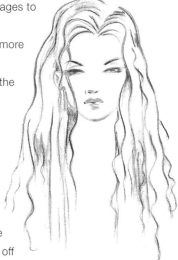

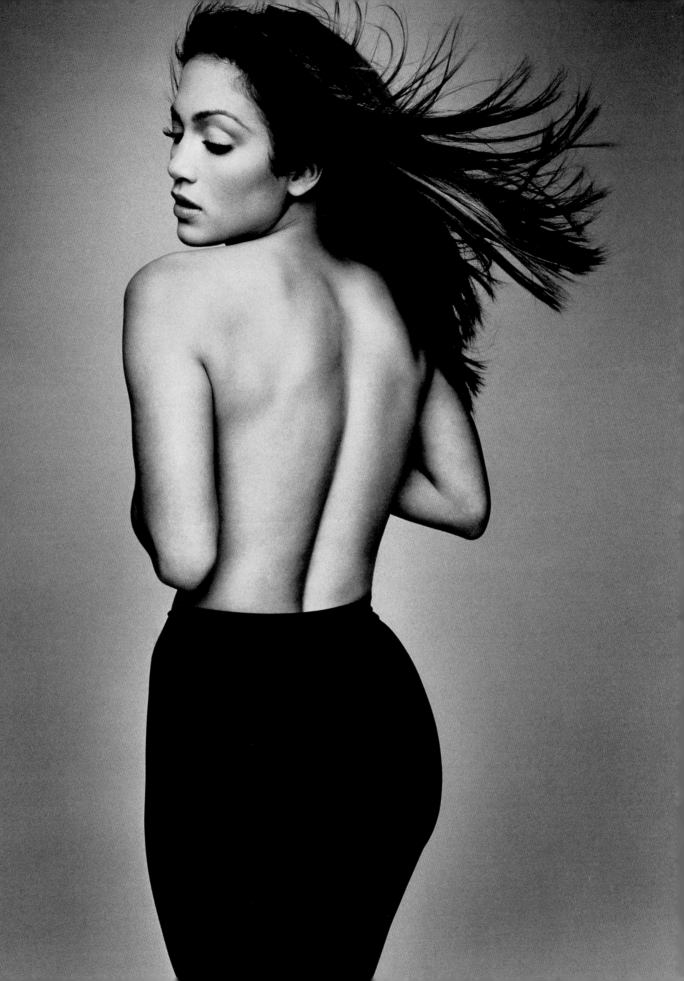

Body Image
y La Vida Buena

WE'VE ALL SEEN HER: *LA GORDITA*. SHE'S WEARING SPANDEX FROM THE NECK DOWN, probably in a shimmery gold color. She's not afraid to shake what her *mami* gave her. When she walks, she flows, and as far as she is concerned, she's looking *good*. Other women might look at her and think, *M'ija*, get out of those hot pants and into the gym. Meanwhile, men look at her and think, *Si cocinas como caminas…*

What's going on here? Frankly, there is something to be learned from that not-exactly-petite, Lycra-encased *muchacha*. Her motto is "I'm not fat, I'm Latina." She's got great T&A. And we could use some of what she's got.

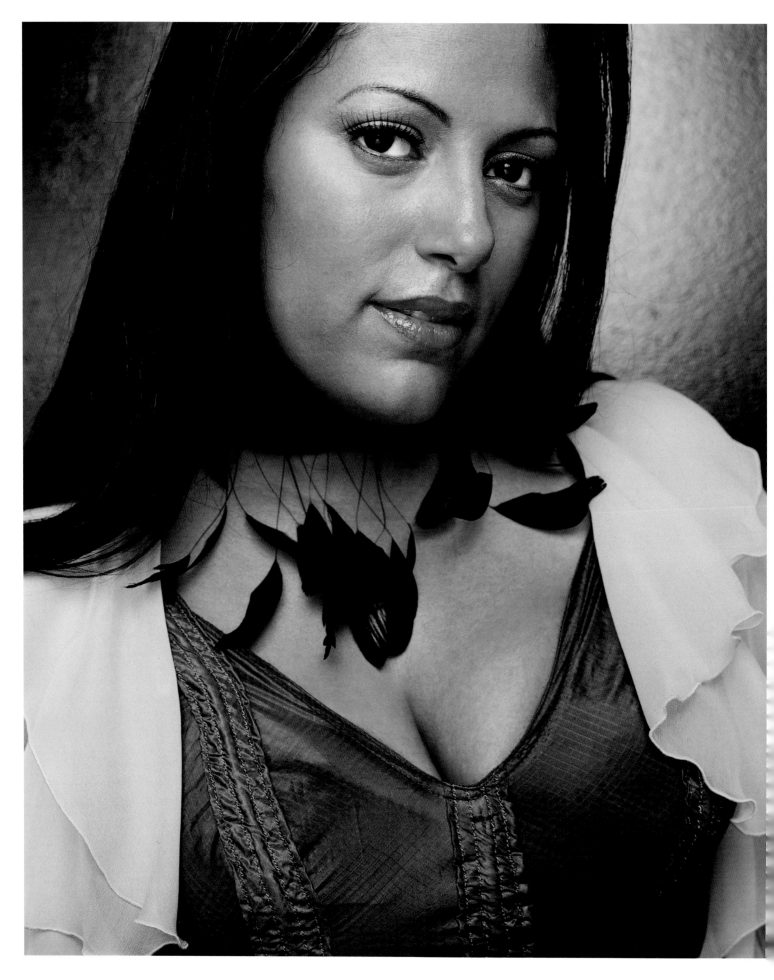

"I'm so happy to be who I am. Physically, I feel great. I've been a size 12 for 10 years or so. I don't listen to Hollywood's definition of what I should be; I'm Cuban American, and my family and friends never had that standpoint. As far as they're concerned, you have to have curves to dance salsa."
—DIANA CHIBAS, PLUS-SIZE MODEL

Behold the Power of **T&A**

TENACITY AND ATTITUDE IS WHAT SHE HAS. CURVACEOUS *COMADRES* know that they are fine the way they are—despite what they weigh or how much they are told by the media that they must get thin, thin, thin. And by wearing what they want and moving like they are just *it*, these women express that attitude loud and proud, doing for body image what Frida Kahlo did for the unibrow.

Traditionally, in our community, there has been nothing wrong with a woman who has a little meat on her bones. In fact, it was encouraged. *Gordita* is a term of endearment. Being "*bien cuidada*" meant being healthy, well fed, and, literally, cared for. We have a history of embracing an image of femininity that is substantive, strong, and sexy.

This doesn't mean our community doesn't have our own complex body issues. While young Caucasian women tended to starve themselves, many less-well-endowed Latinas grew up thinking "skinny" was synonymous with "ugly." Yet a troubling trend is on the rise: Studies show that our perception of the ideal body type changes substantially as we adapt to the culture of the United States. The longer a Hispanic woman has spent time in this country, the more likely she is to have absorbed narrow cultural ideals of beauty.

This trend occurs at the same time that American culture is looking to our community for an alternative image of what is beautiful. Witness the Jennifer Lopez phenomenon—the woman who became as famous for her backside as for her face. Or Salma Hayek, who even at size two is repeatedly featured in stories about the new "voluptuousness." So what is a Latina supposed to think, feel, and perceive about her own body when she is getting so many conflicting messages?

Rita Hayworth (below) had beautiful, natural *curvas* that were all hers. Suzette Quintanilla (right) looks beautiful, glamorous, and— more important—happy.

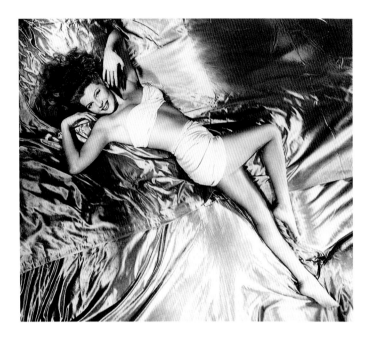

*"My aunts used to say to me,
'A man never thinks, Que lindos huesos.'"*
—LIZ TORRES

Throw out the stereotypes

What the *gordita* with plenty of T&A knows is that trying to fulfill someone else's image of what is beautiful means you will waste a lot of time trying to be something you are not. Body stereotypes abound both within and outside of our community. Take, for example, the idea that being big is OK, but you have to be big in the right places—like the chest, hips, and backside, but not the waist.

Latinas are generalized as being voluptuous, meaning ample breasts and a curvy rear, but a good number of us don't fit this description. This is why stereotypes have no place in the pantheon of Latina beauty. If you take anything from this book, it should be the recognition that our beauty is so diverse, so multifaceted, so amazing in all its many incarnations, that stereotypes simply can't rein us in. Stereotypes are for people with small minds, anyway. People with small minds need easy solutions, consistent images, and a "right" way to be think, be, and act. *La gordita*, with her spandex hot pants, has a mind (and a hip measurement) that is far too expansive to be contained by such a flimsy idea.

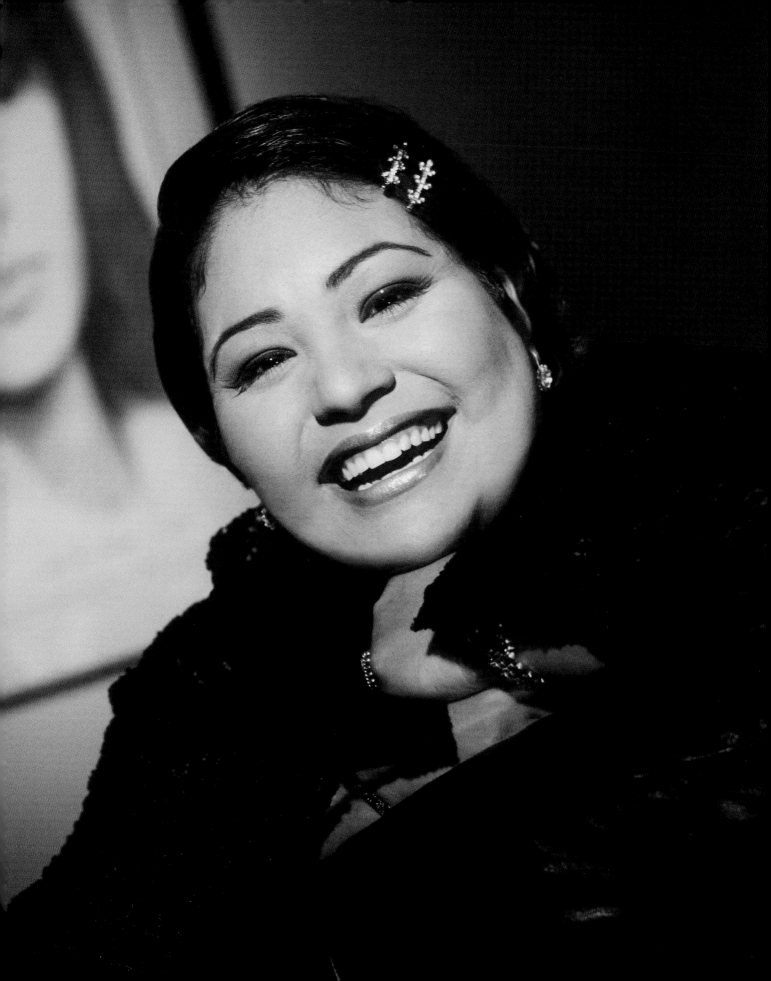

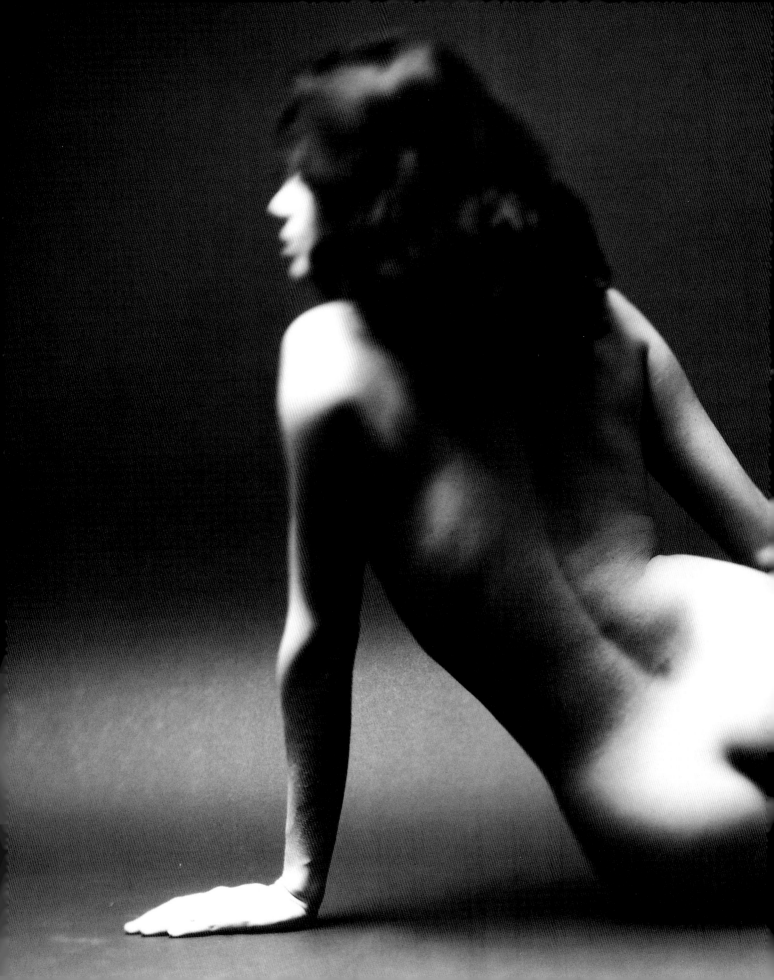

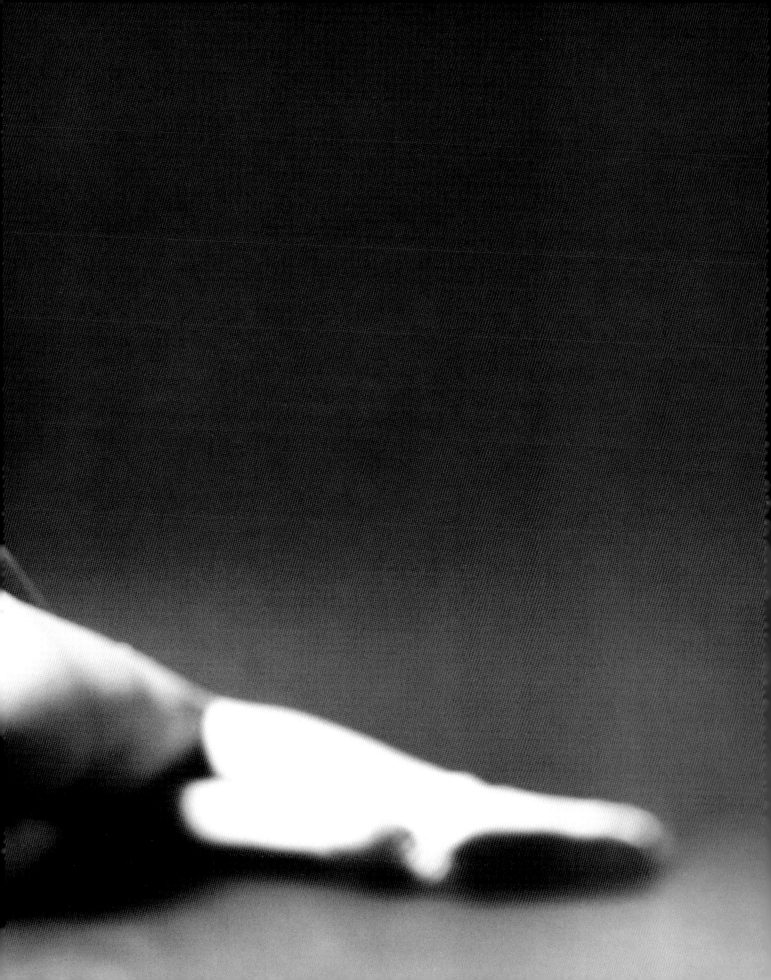

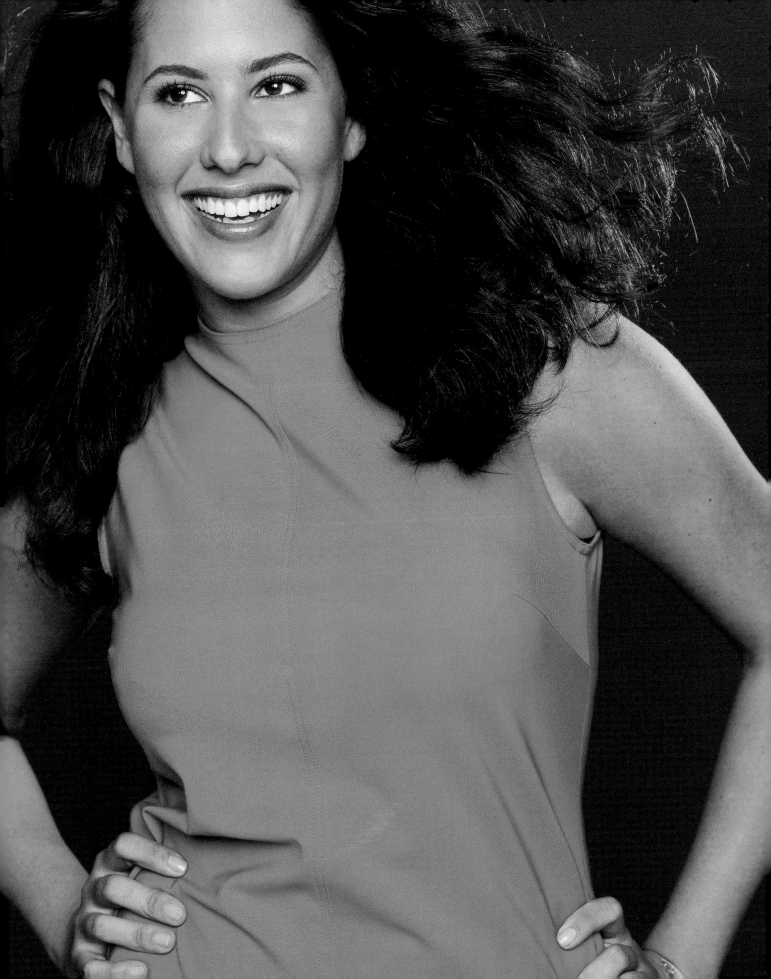

Start the Process

A HEALTHY BODY IMAGE ISN'T A GIVEN—IT'S A PROCESS. IT INVOLVES slowly but surely adapting attitudes toward our bodies that are empowering instead of belittling. It involves making peace with the food we love, and it requires us to take our health seriously.

A healthy body image is a reality you can make yours now, not some far-off, unattainable thing that will happen when you lose or gain another 10 pounds. This confidence enables you to move easily past the inevitable set-backs that come with real life. It makes it OK to have a day when you're not feeling exactly "small-boned." It allows you to enjoy a family feast without PTSS (Post-*Tamales* Stress Syndrome). It affords you the luxury of being human—a human who respects and enjoys her body, loves what it can do, and takes care of it in the best way possible.

As with most accomplishments in life, a healthy body image is born from within. Here are some traits to work toward:

• **Don't be critical of other women's bodies.**

We've all been guilty of this one. But making yourself feel better at the expense of another person only lasts until you see someone else who's better-looking than you—and there are always plenty of them, no matter how beautiful you are. Even the most stunning woman in the world will be acutely aware of the one woman in the room more stunning than she is, even if no one else would agree with that judgment. So stop the madness. And stop comparing your *nalgas* to somebody else's.

• **Have an accurate picture in your head of what you look like.**

Not how you'd like to look. Not how you think you look in your worst night-mare—how you really look. The truth is, an accurate awareness of your size is a key to staying healthy. Anorexics and bulimics both suffer from a disorder that stems from literally being unable to "see" what they look like. They peer into the mirror and see a fat girl when what they are is a very sad girl who is wasting her-self and her life away. Not a pretty picture.

• **Walk with a purpose.**

Posture is a huge indicator of how you feel inside. So command respect and attention with your walk—no hesitancy, timidity, or "I'm feeling so sorry for myself" allowed here. Broadcast to the world that you are in charge, and the world will believe you.

*"It doesn't matter what my body looks like, it's what
my body feels like. That's what my body image is based on.
When I'm loose and limber and graceful I feel like I am beautiful.
It doesn't matter what I look like outwardly."*
—ESMERALDA SANTIAGO

- **Be honest and responsible about when you need to make lifestyle changes.**

Yes, being a *gordita* is fine, but when too much weight slows you down, threatens your health, and makes it hard to complete simple tasks or a challenge to keep up with your kids, it's time for some changes, *pronto*.

- **When it's time to get busy with your *cariño*, you have no problems getting naked.**

Thin women certainly do not have the monopoly on great sex lives. And, as Iris Chacón and Raquel Welch both proved, rail-thin women certainly don't have the monopoly on being sex goddesses, either. So when you are with your *amorcito* and you're both ready to be intimate, your willingness to be uninhibited—in every respect—is a big clue to the state of your body image. When you are thinking about how you are feeling instead of what he is seeing, then you know you are an official sex goddess supreme.

Iris Chacón (below) had a figure that defied the laws of gravity. Rita Moreno (opposite) made moves as a dancer that amazed the world.

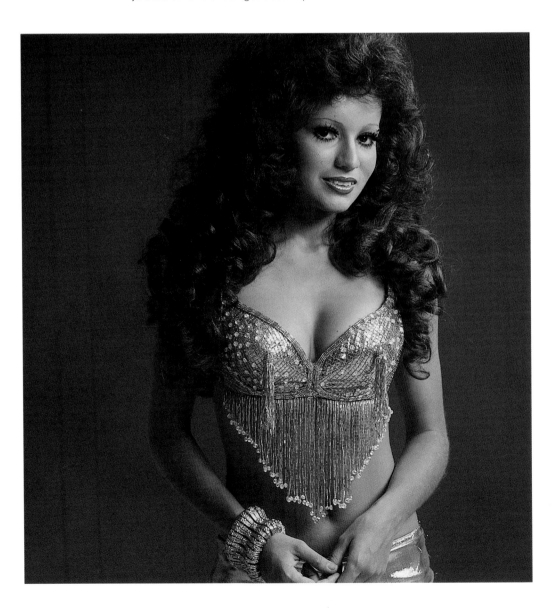

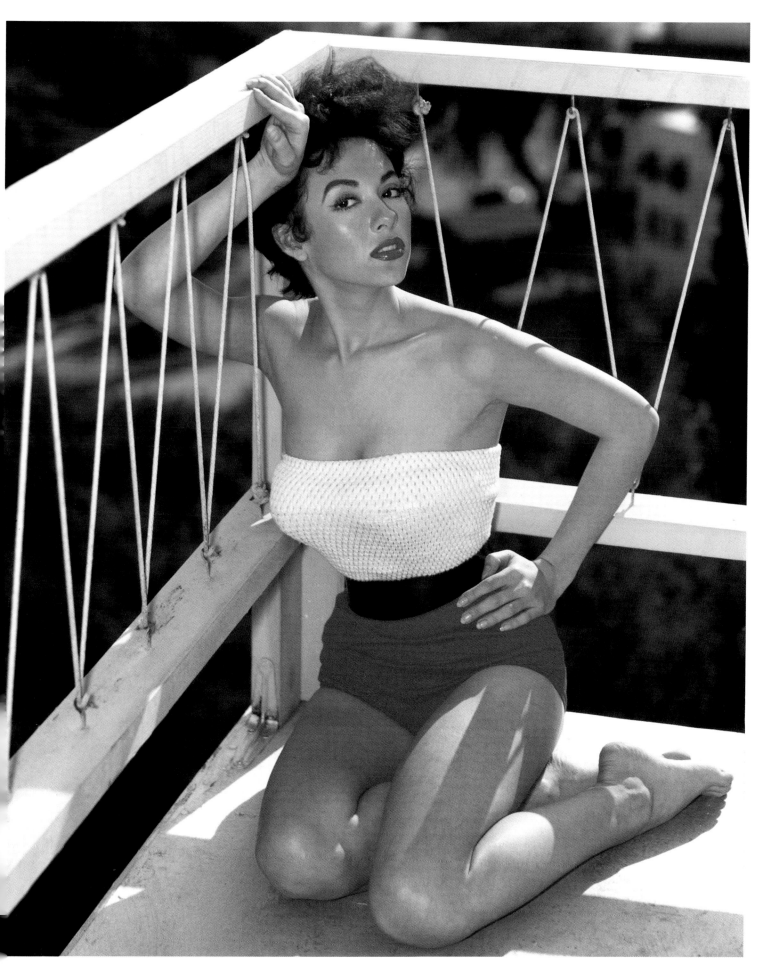

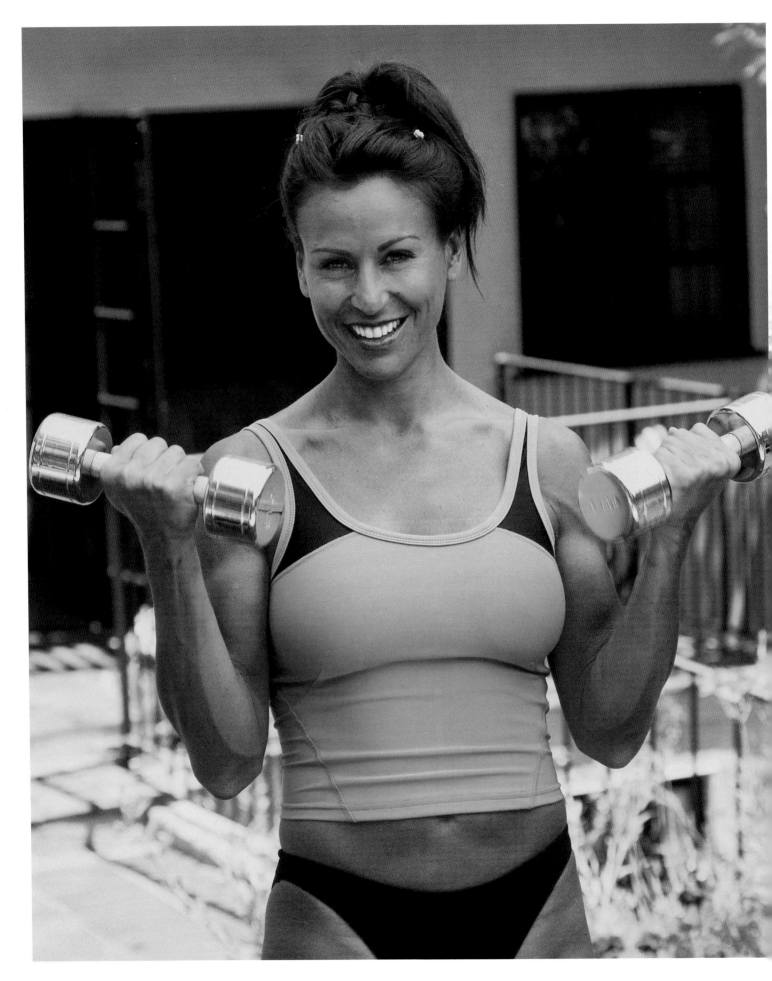

¡Muévelo *Muévelo!*

INCORPORATING EXERCISE INTO YOUR LIFE IS VITAL TO HAVING A healthy body image. Since we know that beautiful doesn't only come in a size six, and we also all know *gorditas* who are strong, fast, and agile enough to kick some serious butt, it's time to look at movement as part of this process.

Exercise's greatest impact is on how you feel. Exercise releases endorphins, the body's own natural painkillers. They are responsible for the lift you feel after having completed a good workout. You owe it to yourself to access these all-natural mood-lifters as much as you can. Instead of saying you can't afford the time, realize that you can't afford not to make the time to move.

● **Get a routine down, then change it.**

Some people enjoy routine. Others can't stand it, in any part of their lives. Whether you are of either extreme or somewhere between the two on the exercise-also-needs-to-entertain-me continuum, you need to create an exercise program that will support your personality. Don't try to force yourself into an aerobics class if what you really want to do is learn to tango.

Another option is to try fit exercise into your lifestyle by making smaller changes: walking more, chasing your kids, or even having more (and more rigorous) sex. Do anything, just make sure it's regular and that you keep your eye on what you would like to learn to do later on.

The human body thrives on change. When your body gets used to a routine and has learned and mastered the new things you were exposing it to, the level of benefits being reaped begins to plateau.

Realizing this can be enormously liberating. It frees us to try new things and learn more about ourselves. The benefits of changing your routine are most evident for people who exercise regularly. When they experiment with a new regimen they read about in a magazine or take a new class and happily report, "It really works! I'm noticing a difference," what they are noticing is how their bodies have been jump-started by a shift in the habitual. Forcing yourself to change brings us to the next point about movement and exercise:

● **Don't be afraid to look silly.**

Being awkward, clumsy, or gawky goes hand-in-hand with learning something new. The thing to fear is doing nothing at all.

● **Pick a goal that exceeds your dress size.**

Climb the pyramids at Teotihuacan. Become an excellent salsa dancer. Go whitewater rafting in Costa Rica. Trek the trails to Macchu Picchu. Activities like these require *cojones* and a ready-to-go level of fitness. So decide what you want. Then get ready to go.

Opposite: Gisselle Fernandez pumps some iron. Whatever you do, whenever you do it, just make a commitment to move.

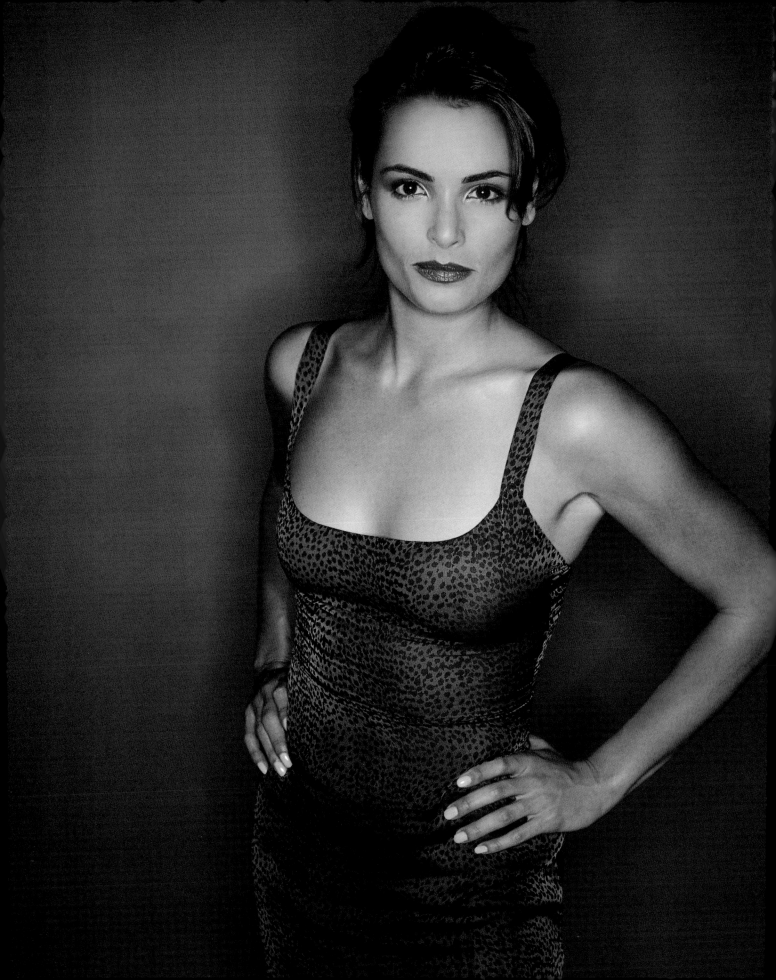

*"I think a healthy love affair can really help
you to stay fit. The other person is making you feel
beautiful and sexy and loved, so you don't need
to stuff yourself with chocolate."*
—LEONORA VARELA

Food, **Glorious** Food

GOD BLESS THE HISPANIC KITCHEN. IT MAKES THE WORLD A MUCH nicer place in which to live. Food is more than fuel in our culture; for us, it's part of our history, our identity, and our families. In fact, the whole notion of "comfort food" probably originated in our culture alongside the pot of beans and rice. We love food. Yet you can't separate your eating patterns from your body image, nor should you try to. Your body reflects what you put in it. While this section is by no means a substitute for the advice of your doctor or a healthy eating plan, here are some basic principles you should try to adapt:

- **Everything in moderation is OK.**
- **Eat at least five servings of fruits and vegetables a day.**
- **Move continuously and vigorously for at least 30 minutes three times a week.**
- **Drink milk for calcium. If you can't stand milk, take supplements.**
- **Don't berate yourself for indulging once in a while.**

As we said before, food is more than food in our community. To try to ignore this by, say, denying yourself a healthy portion of *arroz con pollo* at a family gathering is akin to living a soulless, vacuous, uninspired life. Sound like fun? We don't think so either.

- **Don't follow fad diets.**

One protein-only regime that is hot right now would have us chomping on *chicharrones* 24-7, while depriving us of *pan dulce*. Why would you want to subject yourself to that when you can have your *chicharrones* (once in a while) and eat your *pan dulce*, too?

Loving your body, in the end, means your mind has to be in alignment with your actions—because how you treat your body is a direct reflection of how it looks. *Cuida tus curvas*. Love them as much as you love yourself. And don't stand for anyone—not the media, not your family, not your partner—making you feel like anything other than the strong, sexy, intelligent *mamacita* you are. You are what makes *la vida buena*.

Credits

Acknowledgments

THIS WAS TRULY A GROUP PROJECT THAT WE ARE *ORGULLOSA* TO HAVE BEEN A PART OF.

We'd like to thank Katherine Cowles, the agent for this book, for her original insight into the conspicuous lack of a beauty book for, by, and about Latina women, as well as for her unflagging belief in the project. To Peternelle van Arsdale, who saw the potential in the proposal, and helped to bring the Hyperion team behind this, we thank you very much.

Many thanks to the editors from *Latina* who contributed their time, research and talents. In particular, this book would not have been possible without *Latina*'s gifted art director Irasema Rivera, who drew upon the remarkable images she has created for *Latina* each month to celebrate the many faces of Latina beauty in this book.

Mil gracias also to Laura Encinas who has all the contacts and always gets the *permiso*, and to Maria Collazo for her tireless work to get just the right image of Iris Chacón, Rita Hayworth and Rita Moreno, among others. Deserving of *un gran abrazo* for their research and contributions are Michelle Herrera Mulligan, Ebelinda Antigua, Yesenia Almonte, Yesenia De Avila, Robin Moreno, Anamary Pelayo, Alicia Ruiz, and the Mistress of Information For The Latina Nation, Michelle Longo.

Thanks also go to Welcome—especially *los hermanos* Wakabayashi—who showed us that they, too, believed that Latinas deserve a book that is as beautiful as they are. To their copyeditor Carrie Schneider, thanks for being so quick.

Finally, *muchas gracias* to all the unsung heros: the dermatologists, makeup artists, hairstylists, and specialists who contributed their knowledge to this book—even though they weren't directly quoted! Dr. Hector L. Franco (who gave his time to review an early copy of Chapter 6), Dr. Maritza Perez, Dr. David E. Bank, Elena Avila, Dr. Jane Delgado, Valerie Orlando-Velez, Sherrae, Whitney James, Luis Guillermo, Sonomi Obinata, Dickey, Matthew Vanleeuwen, Linda Shonning, Lillian Marquez, Billy B., Manuela Goncalves, and Dr. Ana Nogales. Thanks to Mario Cáder-Frech for his *Remedios Caseros* in Chapter 6. And finally, a special acknowledgement to Gloria Rodriguez, who served as inspiration for many of the ideas discussed in "You've Got *Ese Algo*."

Your knowledge and experience has meant a great deal to the women who will read and learn from this book, and finally see themselves for the true beauties that they are.

—THE EDITORS OF *LATINA* MAGAZINE AND BELÉN ARANDA-ALVARADO

Produced by Welcome Enterprises, Inc.
Designed by Gregory Wakabayashi

Library of Congress Cataloging-in-Publication Data

Latina beauty / by the editors of Latina magazine and Belén Aranda-Alvarado.
p. cm.
ISBN 0-7868-6669-1
1. Beauty, Personal. 2. Hispanic American women. 3. Face—Care and hygiene.
4. Cosmetics. I. Aranda-Alvarado, Belén. II. Latina magazine.

RA778 .L356 2000
646.7'042'08968073—dc21

00-040760

FIRST EDITION

10 9 8 7 6 5 4 3 2 1

Printed in Japan by Toppan Printing Co. Ltd.